Encyclopedia of Electromyography: Diverse Applications

Volume IV

Encyclopedia of Electromyography: Diverse Applications Volume IV

Edited by **Michael Backman**

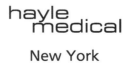

hayle medical

New York

Published by Hayle Medical,
30 West, 37th Street, Suite 612,
New York, NY 10018, USA
www.haylemedical.com

Encyclopedia of Electromyography: Diverse Applications
Volume IV
Edited by Michael Backman

International Standard Book Number: 978-1-63241-162-4 (Hardback)

This book contains information obtained from authentic and highly regarded sources. Copyright for all individual chapters remain with the respective authors as indicated. A wide variety of references are listed. Permission and sources are indicated; for detailed attributions, please refer to the permissions page. Reasonable efforts have been made to publish reliable data and information, but the authors, editors and publisher cannot assume any responsibility for the validity of all materials or the consequences of their use.

The publisher's policy is to use permanent paper from mills that operate a sustainable forestry policy. Furthermore, the publisher ensures that the text paper and cover boards used have met acceptable environmental accreditation standards.

Trademark Notice: Registered trademark of products or corporate names are used only for explanation and identification without intent to infringe.

Printed in the United States of America.

Contents

Preface   VII

EMG Analysis and Applications   1

Chapter 1   **Normalization of EMG Signals: To Normalize or Not to
             Normalize and What to Normalize to?**   3
             Mark Halaki and Karen Ginn

Chapter 2   **Nonlinear Analysis of Surface EMG Signals**   23
             Min Lei and Guang Meng

Chapter 3   **EMG Decomposition and Artefact Removal**   79
             Adriano O. Andrade, Alcimar B. Soares,
             Slawomir J. Nasuto and Peter J. Kyberd

Chapter 4   **Sphincter EMG for Diagnosing Multiple System
             Atrophy and Related Disorders**   105
             Ryuji Sakakibara, Tomoyuki Uchiyama, Tatsuya Yamamoto, Fuyuki
             Tateno, Tomonori Yamanishi, Masahiko Kishi and Yohei Tsuyusaki

Chapter 5   **The Usefulness of Mean and Median
             Frequencies in Electromyography Analysis**   125
             Angkoon Phinyomark, Sirinee Thongpanja, Huosheng Hu,
             Pornchai Phukpattaranont and Chusak Limsakul

Chapter 6   **Feature Extraction Methods for Studying Surface
             Electromyography and Kinematic Measurements
             in Parkinson's Disease**   151
             Saara M. Rissanen, Markku Kankaanpää,
             Mika P. Tarvainen and Pasi A. Karjalainen

Chapter 7   **Distinction of Abnormality of Surgical Operation
             on the Basis of Surface EMG Signals**   177
             Chiharu Ishii

Permissions

List of Contributors

Preface

This book has been an outcome of determined endeavour from a group of educationists in the field. The primary objective was to involve a broad spectrum of professionals from diverse cultural background involved in the field for developing new researches. The book not only targets students but also scholars pursuing higher research for further enhancement of the theoretical and practical applications of the subject.

Electromyography (EMG) is a technique for evaluating and recording the electrical activity produced by skeletal muscles. EMG is used for the diagnosis of neuromuscular issues and for determining biomechanical and motor control deficiency and other functional disorders. Moreover, it can be applied as a control signal for interfacing with orthotic and/or prosthetic devices or other rehabilitation aids. This book covers the current diverse applications applied in EMG research. It will provide readers with a comprehensive introduction to EMG signal processing techniques and applications, while presenting several new results and explanation of existing algorithms.

It was an honour to edit such a profound book and also a challenging task to compile and examine all the relevant data for accuracy and originality. I wish to acknowledge the efforts of the contributors for submitting such brilliant and diverse chapters in the field and for endlessly working for the completion of the book. Last, but not the least; I thank my family for being a constant source of support in all my research endeavours.

Editor

EMG Analysis and Applications

Normalization of EMG Signals: To Normalize or Not to Normalize and What to Normalize to?

Mark Halaki and Karen Ginn

Additional information is available at the end of the chapter

1. Introduction

Electromyography (EMG) has been around since the 1600s [1]. It is a tool used to measure the action potentials of motor units in muscles [2]. The EMG electrodes are like little microphones which "listen" for muscle action potentials so having these microphones in different locations relative to the muscle or motor units affects the nature of the recording [3]. The amplitude and frequency characteristics of the raw electromyogram signal have been shown to be highly variable and sensitive to many factors. De Luca [4] provided a detailed account of these characteristics which have a "basic" or "elemental" effect on the signal dividing them into extrinsic and intrinsic sub-factors. Extrinsic factors are those which can be influenced by the experimenter, and include: electrode configuration (distance between electrodes as well as area and shape of the electrodes); electrode placement with respect to the motor points in the muscle and lateral edge of the muscle as well as the orientation to the muscle fibres; skin preparation and impedance [5, 6]; and perspiration and temperature [7]. Intrinsic factors include: physiological, anatomical and biochemical characteristics of the muscles such as the number of active motor units; fiber type composition of the muscles; blood flow in the muscle; muscle fiber diameter; the distance between the active fibers within the muscle with respect to the electrode; and the amount of tissue between the surface of the muscle and the electrode. These factors vary between individuals, between days within an individual and within a day in an individual if the electrode set up has been altered. Given that there are many factors that influence the EMG signal, voltage recorded from a muscle is difficult to describe in terms of level if there is no reference value to which it can be compared. Therefore, interpretation of the amplitude of the raw EMG signal is problematic unless some kind of normalization procedure is performed. Normalization refers to the conversion of the signal to a scale relative to a known and repeatable value. It has been reported [8] that normalized EMG signals were first presented by Eberhart, Inman & Bresler in 1954 [9]. Since then, there have been a number of methods used to normalize EMG signals with no consensus as to which method is most appropriate [8]. In this chapter, we will outline when the presentation of raw EMG is acceptable and when normalization is essential as well as the various methods used to normalize EMG signals. A discussion of the advantages and disadvantages of each method and examples of its uses will be provided.

2. Raw EMG signals (without normalization)

As indicated in the introduction, there are many factors that influence the EMG signal. However, it is generally accepted that within a data collection session and within an individual where no changes have been made to the configuration of the EMG set-up (electrode placement, amplification, filtering etc), under constant temperature and humidity conditions and within a short period of time, the raw EMG can be used for limited comparisons such as:

1. the analysis of the frequency content of the EMG signal. In this type of analysis, the power spectrum of the EMG signal can be obtained by applying a Fast Fourier Transform to the EMG signal. The power density function of the EMG provides a distribution of the signal power as a function of frequency. Changes in the shape of the power density function of the EMG is usually analysed and shifts in the power density to lower frequencies is associated with fatigue. Since the shape of the power spectra is what is important, the amplitude of the EMG signal is not critical and EMG normalization is not required.
2. the decomposition of the EMG into wavelets for an analysis of motor unit firing patterns, or cross talk between muscles. In this analysis, the EMG signal is decomposed into small wavelets (small waveforms). The wavelets are then used to identify and characterize motor unit action potentials by compressing and/or rescaling the wavelets and identifying them in the EMG signal. Again, the amplitude of the EMG signal is not critical and EMG normalization is not required.
3. the time of the initiation of muscle activation. This type of analysis does not require EMG normalization as the time of activation is usually identified from the raw signal e.g. when the raw EMG signal amplitude reaches 2 [10] or 3 [11] standard deviations of the mean above baseline levels.
4. amplitude comparisons of signals from a given muscle between short term interventions/movements within an individual in the same session under the same experimental conditions without changes to the EMG electrode set-up [12] e.g. when comparing the EMG signal between different interventions/movements in a given muscle in each individual [13-16]. Because the absolute amplitude of the signal is meaningless, one cannot evaluate the level of activity in the muscle, but only that it is more or less active in one intervention/movement compared to the other. Therefore, comparison of muscle activity levels between muscles or individuals is not valid.

3. Normalization of EMG signals

To be able to compare EMG activity in the same muscle on different days or in different individuals or to compare EMG activity between muscles, the EMG must be normalized [4,

17, 18]. Normalization of EMG signals is usually performed by dividing the EMG signals during a task by a reference EMG value obtained from the same muscle. By normalizing to a reference EMG value collected using the same electrode configuration, factors that affect the EMG signals during the task and the reference contraction are the same. Therefore, one can validly obtain a relative measure of the activation compared to the reference value.

The common consensus is that a "good" reference value to which to normalize EMG signals should have high repeatability, especially in the same subject in the same session, and be meaningful. By choosing a reference value repeatable within an individual, one can compare the levels obtained from any task to that reference value. The choice of reference value should allow comparisons between individuals and between muscles. To be able to do so, the reference value should have similar meaning between individuals and between muscles. The choice of normalization method is critical in the interpretation of the EMG signals as it will influence the amplitude and pattern of the EMG signals [8]. Unfortunately, there is no consensus as to a single "best" method for normalization of EMG data [8, 18] and a variety of methods have been used to obtain normalization reference values:

1. Maximum (peak) activation levels during maximum contractions
2. Peak or mean activation levels obtained during the task under investigation
3. Activation levels during submaximal isometric contractions
4. Peak to peak amplitude of the maximum M-wave (M-max)

3.1. Maximum (peak) activation levels during maximum contractions

3.1.1. Maximal voluntary isometric contractions

The most common method of normalizing EMG signals from a given muscle uses to the EMG recorded from the same muscle during a maximal voluntary isometric contraction (MVIC) as the reference value [19-23]. The process of normalization using MVICs is that a reference test (usually a manual muscle test) is identified which produces a maximum contraction in the muscle of interest. Based on the repeatability between tests measures, it is recommended that at least 3 repetitions of the test be performed separated by at least 2 minutes to reduce any fatigue effects [12]. The EMG signals are then processed either by high-pass filtering, rectifying and smoothing or by calculating the root mean square of the signal. The maximum value obtained [12] from the processed signals during all repetitions of the test is then used as the reference value for normalizing the EMG signals, processed in the same way, from the muscle of interest. This allows the assessment of the level of activity of the muscle of interest during the task under investigation compared to the maximal neural activation capacity of the muscle [24-26].

This method sounds simple enough. However, when trying to implement it, investigators are faced with an important question: *What test should be used to produce maximum neural activation in a given muscle?* The choice of MVIC should reflect the maximal neural activation capacity of the given muscle [27]. Unfortunately, there is no consensus as to which test produces maximal activation in all individuals in any given muscle. Table 1 provides some examples of different tests that have been used for the same muscle in different studies. Note the number of different reference tests used for each muscle indicating the lack of consensus as to what test generates maximum activity in any given muscle.

Muscles investigated	Manual muscle test
upper trapezius	• shoulder shrug [28, 29] • combined shoulder elevation/arm flexion/abduction in the scapular plane at 90° abduction [30] • shoulder abduction in scapular plane at 90° abduction [31, 32] • lumbar extension [33]
supraspinatus	• shoulder abduction at 90°, internal rotation (seated) [28] • shoulder abduction at 90°, elbow flexed to 90° (seated) [34] • shoulder external rotation and abduction, shoulder abducted to 20°, elbow flexed to 90°, no shoulder flexion [29]
infraspinatus	• shoulder external rotation, arm at side, elbow flexed to 90° (seated) [28, 31, 34] • shoulder external rotation, shoulder abducted to 45°, elbow flexed to 90°, no shoulder flexion [29]
subscapularis	• shoulder internal rotation, arm at side, elbow flexed to 90° (seated) [28, 34] • shoulder internal rotation, shoulder abducted to 45°, elbow flexed to 90°, no shoulder flexion [29]
latissimus dorsi	• shoulder depression with resistance or adduction and internal rotation, arm at side (seated) [28] • shoulder extension and internal rotation with arm straight, abducted to 30° in the coronal plane and internally rotated [29] • shoulder extension (prone lying) [35, 36]
serratus anterior	• scapular protraction, shoulder abducted to 90°-100° (seated) [28] • scapular protraction, elbow flexed to 45°, shoulder abducted to 75° and internally rotated to 45° [29]
upper rectus abdominis	• trunk flexion, hips and knees flexed to 90°, feet supported, trunk in full flexion (supine) [35, 36] • trunk flexion, legs bent at 45°,and secured, trunk position not mentioned (supine) [37]
internal oblique	• trunk flexion and lateral flexion, hips and knees flexed to 90°, feet supported, trunk in full flexion and rotated contra-laterally (supine) [35] • trunk flexion and lateral flexion, hips and knees flexed to 90°, feet supported, trunk in full flexion and rotated ipsi-laterally (supine) [36]
gluteus maximus	• hip extension, hip flexed 45° (prone) [38] • back extension, hip flexed 30° (seated) [39] • hip abduction at 10° abduction, leg fully extended (side lying) contra-lateral knee and hip flexed 30° [40]
gluteus medius	• hip abduction at 10° abduction, leg fully extended (side lying) contra-lateral knee and hip flexed 30° [40, 41] • hip abduction at 25° abduction, leg fully extended (side lying) [42]

Muscles investigated	Manual muscle test
vastus lateralis	• knee extension, knee flexed 90°, hip flexed 90° (sitting) [38, 43] • knee extension, knee flexed 60°, hip flexed 90° (sitting) [44, 45] • knee extension, knee flexed 45° (sitting) [37]
vastus medialis	• knee extension, knee flexed 60° (sitting) [44, 45] • knee extension, knee flexed 90°, hip flexed 90° (sitting) [43]
rectus femoris	• knee extension, knee flexed 90°, hip flexed 80° to 90° (sitting) [35, 36, 38, 43] • knee extension, knee flexed 60°, hip flexed 90° (sitting) [44-46]
lateral hamstring (biceps femoris) long head	• knee flexion, knee flexed 90°, hip flexed 90° (sitting) [38] • knee flexion, knee flexed 60° (sitting) [44, 46] • knee flexion, knee flexed 60° (prone) [45] • knee flexion, knee flexed 90°, hands clasped behind head (prone) [37]
gastrocnemius lateralis	• ankle plantar flexion, ankle -15°, knee flexed 30° [44] • ankle plantar flexion, mid ankle position (standing unilateral – body weight) [47] • ankle plantar flexion, ankle, knee and hip in neutral position (prone) [45]
gastrocnemius medialis	• ankle plantar flexion, ankle, knee and hip in neutral position (prone) [38, 45] • ankle plantar flexion, ankle -15°, knee flexed 30° [44] • ankle plantar flexion, mid ankle position (standing unilateral – body weight) [47] • ankle plantar flexion (supine) [33]
soleus	• ankle plantar flexion, mid ankle position (prone) [38] • ankle plantar flexion, ankle in neutral position; knee and hip flexed 90° (quadruped position) [45, 46]
tibialis anterior	• ankle dorsi flexion, ankle, knee and hip in neutral position (supine) [45] • ankle dorsi flexion, ankle in neutral position; knee and hip flexed 90° (quadruped position) [46]

Table 1. Examples of MVIC tests used to generate maximum activity levels in various muscles

Although the repeatability of the EMG recorded during MVICs within individuals on the same day has been questioned [34], the majority of studies indicate that the reliability of MVICs within individuals on the same day is high [42, 48, 49]. High repeatability requires proper guidance of the subjects to perform the tests identically with each repetition, familiarity of the subjects with the production of maximum effort and the avoidance of fatigue.

Because the test that will yield maximal activation in any given muscle is not known, many studies report EMG levels during various tasks that are >100% MVIC particularly during rapid, forceful contractions [18] or eccentric contractions [50]. For example, Jobe et al. [51] reported EMG signals from serratus anterior and triceps brachii during the acceleration phase of the over arm throw to be 226% and 212% respectively of the EMG from maximal manual muscle tests which were not described. Reported normalized EMG signals >100% indicate that the normalization test used to generate the MVIC is not accurately revealing the maximum muscle activation capacity. If maximum activity in each muscle is not obtained during the normalization contractions, a systematic error will be introduced which leads to an over estimation of activation levels [30]. This could lead to an incorrect interpretation of the intensity of the muscle activity required to perform a given task. In addition, if the activity in all muscles is not being referenced to the same activity level, e.g. maximum capacity, comparison of activity levels between muscles is not valid.

The problem of not eliciting maximum capacity in each muscle tested would be avoided if standard tests that reliably elicit maximum activation levels were identified [52]. A number of studies have attempted to identify voluntary isometric tests that produce maximum activation levels in various muscles. These studies have shown that multiple tests can produce maximum recording from any given muscle [52-56] and that no specific test produces maximum recording from a given muscle in all individuals tested [27, 53, 54, 56-63]. These findings indicate that the use of single MVIC test to identify maximum activity in a given muscle is not valid and that sets of tests are required in order to ensure maximum activity in a given muscle is recorded from all subjects. Table 2 summarizes the sets of MVIC tests that have been shown to produce maximum activity in face, trunk, shoulder and leg muscles.

Provided that maximum neural activation is achieved in all muscles and individuals tested, using MVICs is a highly reliable method to normalize EMG data and can be used to compare activity between muscles, between tasks and between individuals. To achieve the maximum neural activation in all muscles and individuals, sets of MVIC tests that produce maximum activation in each muscle need to be identified. The highest value recorded for each muscle from at least 3 attempts at these MVIC tests should be used as the normalization value to ensure that the recorded values reflect maximum neural activation levels.

Study	Muscles investigated	MVIC test	Isometric tests that produce maximum EMG in the muscles investigated
O'Dwyer et al (1981) [56]	levator labii superiori zygomaticus major buccinator risorius orbicularis oris superioris orbicularis oris inferioris depressor anguli oris depressor labii inferioris mentalis intrinsic tongue muscles anterior genioglossus styloglossus/hyoglossus geniohyoid mylohyoid digastric (anterior belly) internal (medial) pterygoid temporalis	Maximum EMG from each muscle across all tests	1. unilateral snarl 2. broad laugh 3. puff out cheeks, mouth closed 4. broad smile, mouth closed 5. compress upper lip against upper incisors 6. compress lower lip against lower incisors 7. depress comers of mouth 8. depress lower lip, jaw closed 9. raise and evert lower lip while wrinkling chin 10. curl sides of tongue up 11. saliva swallow 12. gentle tongue protrusion 13. lower jaw against resistance 14. intercuspal bite on hard object 15. clench jaw.

Study	Muscles investigated	MVIC test	Isometric tests that produce maximum EMG in the muscles investigated
McGill (1991) [59]	rectus abdominis external oblique internal oblique latissimus dorsi upper erector spinae (T9) lower erector spinae (L3)	1,2,6,7 1,2,5,6,7 1,3,5,6,7 2,3,6,7 3,4,7 4	1. resisted bent-knee sit-up (feet restrained trunk at 30º hands behind head). 2. standing pelvis fixed flexing forward 3. standing pelvis fixed lateral bend 4. hanging over the edge of the test table in a prone posture and extending upward against resistance 5. hanging over the edge of the test table supine and flexing upward against resistance 6. hanging over the edge of the test table on side and lateral bending upward against resistance 7. clockwise and anticlockwise trunk twist at 0º and pre-rotated at ± 30º
Nieminen et al (1993) [61]	supraspinatus infraspinatus upper trapezius middle trapezius lower trapezius anterior deltoid middle deltoid pectoralis major	5,6,7,8 2,5,6,7 5,6,7,8 2,3,4,6,7 1,2,5,6,8 3,5,6,7 2,3,5,6,7 1,4,5,9	1. internal rotation shoulder at 0º abduction, elbow at 90º flexion 2. external rotation shoulder at 0º abduction, elbow at 90º flexion 3. abduction shoulder at 0º abduction 4. shoulder elevation 5. flexion arm horizontal 6. flexion hand 25 cm above and 25 cm right of horizontal 7. flexion hand 25 cm above and 25 cm left of horizontal 8. flexion hand 25 cm below and 25 cm right of horizontal 9. flexion hand 25 cm below and 25 cm left of horizontal
Kelly et al 1996 [54]	supraspinatus infraspinatus subscapularis anterior deltoid middle deltoid posterior deltoid latissimus dorsi pectoralis major	7-9,12-14 10-12 16,17 1-9 7 12 16,17 15	Coded: Activity at shoulder abduction angle; humeral rotation angle 1. abduction at 0º; -45º 2. abduction at 0º; 0º 3. abduction at 0º; +45º 4. abduction at 45º; -45º 5. abduction at 45º; 0º 6. abduction at 45º; +45º 7. abduction at 90º; -45º 8. abduction at 90º; 0º 9. abduction at 90º; +45º 10. external rotation at 0º; -45º 11. external rotation at 45º; -45º 12. external rotation at 90º; -45º 13. external rotation at 90º; 0º 14. external rotation at 90º; +45º 15. internal rotation at 0º; 0º 16. internal rotation at 90º; -45º 17. internal rotation at 90º; 0º

Study	Muscles investigated	MVIC test	Isometric tests that produce maximum EMG in the muscles investigated
Ekstrom et al (2005) [27]	upper trapezius middle trapezius lower trapezius serratus anterior	1,2,3,4,5,7 5,6,7 1,2,3,5,7,8 1,2,3	1. shoulder flexion at 125º with scapula resistance 2. shoulder abducted to 125º scapular plane 3. shoulder abducted to 90º with the neck side bent, rotated to the opposite side, and extended 4. scapula elevated with the neck side bent, rotated to the opposite side, and extended 5. shoulder horizontally abducted and externally rotated 6. shoulder horizontally abducted and internally rotated 7. arm raised above the head in line with the lower trapezius muscle 8. shoulder externally rotated at 90º abduction
Hsu et al (2006) [45]	tibialis anterior lateral gastrocnemius medial gastrocnemius soleus vastus lateralis vastus medialis rectus femoris lateral hamstrings (biceps femoris) medial hamstrings (semitendinosus)	Maximum EMG from each muscle across all tests	1. entire leg flexion and extension, seated with backrest reclined 45º, hip flexed 110º, knee flexed 60º, ankle neutral. 2. knee flexion and extension, seated with backrest vertical, knee flexed 60º
Boettcher et al 2008 [53] and Ginn et al 2011 [57]	supraspinatus infraspinatus subscapularis lower subscapularis upper trapezius middle trapezius lower trapezius serratus anterior latissimus dorsi rhomboid major teres major anterior deltoid middle deltoid posterior deltoid pectoralis major (clavicular head)	Maximum EMG from each muscle across all 5 tests provides >95% chance of eliciting maximum for all muscles	1. shoulder extension seated with the arm at 30º abduction, elbow fully extended, and thumb toward the body; arm extended as resistance applied over the distal forearm. 2. shoulder abduction at 90º with internal rotation 3. shoulder internal rotation in 90º abduction 4. shoulder flexion at 125º with scapula resistance 5. shoulder horizontal adduction at 90º flexion
Chopp et al (2010) [52]	anterior deltoid middle deltoid pectoralis major (clavicular head) pectoralis major (sternal head)	1,4-6,10 2-6 7-12 7,8,10	1. Coded: force direction – shoulder flexion angle – horizontal abduction angle 2. UP-45-0 3. UP-45-45 4. UP-45-90 5. UP-90-0 6. UP-90-45 7. UP-90-90

Study	Muscles investigated	MVIC test	Isometric tests that produce maximum EMG in the muscles investigated
			8. IN-45-0
			9. IN-45-45
			10. IN-45-90
			11. IN-90-0
			12. IN-90-45
			13. IN-90-90
Vera-Garcia et al (2010) [64]	upper rectus abdominis	1,2,6	1. upper trunk flexion
	lower rectus abdominis	1,2,3,4	2. lower trunk flexion
	lateral external oblique	1,3,4,5,6,10	3. upper trunk twisting
	medial external oblique	1,3,5,6	4. lower trunk twisting
	internal oblique	2,3,5,6	5. upper trunk bending
	latissimus dorsi (T9)	3,4,5,9	6. lower trunk bending
	erector spinae (T9)	7,8,9	7. upper trunk extension
	erector spinae (L5)	7,8	8. lower trunk extension
			9. shoulder rotation and adduction
			10. abdominal hollowing
Rutherford et al (2011) [58]	lateral gastrocnemius	2,4,5,6,7,8	1. knee extension at 45º knee flexion in sitting
	medial gastrocnemius	4,5,6,7,8	2. combined knee extension + hip flexion at 45º knee flexion in sitting
	vastus lateralis	1,2,3,7,8	3. knee extension at 15º knee flexion in supine position
	vastus medialis	1,2,3,7,8	
	rectus femoris	1,2,3	4. knee flexion at 15º knee flexion in supine position
	lateral hamstrings (biceps femoris)	4,5,6	5. knee flexion at 55º knee flexion in sitting
	medial hamstrings (semitendinosus)	4,5,6	6. knee flexion at 55º knee flexion in prone position
			7. plantar-flexion at neutral ankle, knee and hip in supine position
			8. unilateral plantar-flexion in standing

Table 2. Examples of studies that have identified tests that produce maximum recordings from given muscles and recommend the use of multiple tests to make sure maximum activation is produced by all individuals tested.

3.1.2. The maximum activation obtained during the task under investigation performed at maximum effort

To reduce the possibility of obtaining normalized EMG levels during a task greater than 100%, investigators have used the EMG obtained during the task under investigation performed at maximum effort as the normalization value. For example, maximum EMG recorded during isometric shoulder abduction has been used to normalize the EMG during submaximal abduction [65], maximum crunch exercise for submaximal crunch exercise [66], maximum sprinting for normalizing the EMG during walking [44, 67] and maximum sprint cycling for normalizing the EMG during cycling [38].

This method of normalizing EMG data produces high reliability between trials [44, 67] and greatly reduces the possibility of obtaining EMG levels during the task of interest greater than the reference value. However, the maximum activation levels of muscles are unknown since maximum force production during the task under investigation does not necessarily produce a maximum activation level in any of the muscles under investigation [8]. In addition, different individuals may use different muscle control strategies to produce the same movement, resulting in different activation levels during the reference contraction in a given muscle between individuals. Therefore, although highly reliable, the use of this method to normalize EMG data to compare muscle activation levels between individuals and between muscles in the task being investigated is not valid. In addition, because this reference value is task dependent, it cannot be used to compare muscle activation levels between different tasks.

3.1.3. The maximum activation obtained at a range of joint angles under maximum effort during dynamic contraction

There is a debate about whether isometric contraction can be used to obtain reference EMG levels for use during dynamic tasks [25]. Some research has found that the EMG levels change with muscle length [68-71], while other studies indicate that joint angle has little effect on maximum EMG levels [72-74] or that there is no consistent pattern of change in the EMG levels with joint angle [74-76]. To address this potential problem, it has been recommended that maximum dynamic (usually isokinetic) contractions be used to obtain reference EMG levels in order to normalize EMG data obtained during movement [77]. In this method, the individual performs a maximum isokinetic contraction at a speed similar to the dynamic task under investigation. The activation levels vs joint angle curve generated from the maximum dynamic contraction is then used to normalize the EMG data [77].

This normalization method has been shown to have low within subject reliability [78] and, because EMG is depended on the velocity of movement for a given force level [79], normalization curves need to be generated for different speeds of movement.

The use of supramaximal stimulation to determine if voluntary contractions are being performed at maximum levels

Maximal voluntary activation can be assessed by interpolation of an electrical stimulus to all or part of the nerve supply to a muscle during maximum voluntary effort. Single electrical stimuli are delivered to the nerve that innervates the muscle during maximum voluntary contraction with increasing intensity until no additional increment in force can be seen. Then 2-4 electric stimuli trains (20 ms between stimuli) are delivered at that intensity as they produce substantially larger evoked responses [80-82]. If the stimulus fails to evoke an increment in force it can be deduced that all motoneurones innervating the muscle are recruited i.e. that the muscle is being maximally activated [83-85].

One criticism of this method of generating maximal activation in a given muscle is that the force output of a muscle during a synchronous activation of the motor neurons, due to the stimulation of a nerve, does not necessarily produce the same force as when the motor neurons are being asynchronously activated by the central nervous system [4].In addition, its use for some muscles will be problematic due to difficulty accessing the nerve/s supplying these muscles e.g. branches of the brachial plexus supplying shoulder muscles. It also has the disadvantage that strong contractions maintained for more than a few seconds will lead to muscle fatigue.

3.2. Peak or mean activation levels obtained during the task under investigation

The first report of normalized EMG signals [9] presented quadriceps EMG signals during walking as a percentage of the peak muscle activity that occurred during the gait cycle [8]. Since then, this method has been used to investigate muscle activation patterns during various activities e.g. walking [25, 86], cycling [87], biceps curl exercise [24] and kayaking [88]. In this method, the EMG data is normalized to the peak or mean activity obtained during the activity in each muscle for each individual separately.

Normalising to the peak or mean amplitude during the activity of interest has been shown to decrease the variability between individuals compared to using raw EMG data or when normalising to MVICs [24, 25, 86, 87]. Normalizing to the mean amplitude during the activity of interest has been reported to be either comparable to [34], or better than [24, 42, 89, 90], normalizing to the peak amplitude during the activity in reducing the variability between subjects. Although the within subject and within day reliability have been shown to be high for both peak and mean amplitude during an activity [42], it has also been shown that they may be less reliable between days in the same individuals compared to normalizing to MVICs [90].

However, the reduction in the variability between individuals by normalising to the peak or mean amplitude recorded during an activity is achieved by removing some real biological variation (e.g. strength difference) between individuals [24, 90]. The amount of muscle activity required to lift a given load, would vary according to each individual's strength. As the reference value used in this method is relative to the task and not to the maximum capacity of the muscle, muscle activity levels cannot be compared between muscles, tasks or individuals. This method, however, can be used to compare patterns of muscle activation between individuals over time [24, 25, 42, 90].

3.3. Activation levels during submaximal isometric contractions

The use of maximal contractions to obtain reference EMG levels has been questioned because of difficulty in getting subjects to mobilize their maximal potential especially in symptomatic subjects who cannot perform a maximum contraction because of pain, muscle inhibition [42, 91] or risk of injury [91]. As a result, the use of tests at submaximal contraction levels have been used to produce reference EMG levels for the purposes of normalizing the EMG signals. De Luca [4] encouraged the use of EMGs from contractions < 80% of MVIC. However, there is no consensus as to whether submaximal contractions have higher within-day reliability than [23], or similar reliability to [92], maximal contractions. Commonly used submaximal isometric contractions include holding a limb against gravity [24, 26, 48, 87, 92] or holding a given load, either an absolute load [24, 93-95] or a relative load determined as a percentage of each individual's maximum load [25]. The muscle activity recorded during the submaximal isometric contraction is then used to normalize the EMG in the same muscle while performing the task under investigation.

The main limitation of using submaximal isometric contractions is that comparisons of activity levels between muscles and individuals are not valid because, once again, the reference value used in this method is not relative to the maximum capacity of the muscle. Lifting an absolute load of say 1 kg mass might require 10% of the maximum muscle capacity in a strong individual compared to say 40% of the maximum muscle capacity in another person who is not as strong. It is not possible to estimate maximum muscle activity from a relative submaximal contraction by linear extrapolation because the torque/EMG relationship is nonlinear [96]. Additionally, the lengths of muscle moment arms in individuals vary and since the EMG signal is related to the force produced by the muscle and not the torque produced by the limb, the force required by the muscle to produce a given torque would be different between individuals. Another limitation is that the motor strategy may not be the same between individuals or between sides within the same individual [95] during the reference submaximal contraction. This is not a problem during maximal contractions as heightened central drive engages all possible muscle resources to achieve the maximum force possible. Therefore, using submaximal isometric contractions as the reference for normalizing EMG data is reliable but doesn't allow valid comparisons between muscles or individuals.

3.4. Peak to peak amplitude of the maximum M-wave (M-max)

This method of normalizing EMG signals involves external stimulation of α-motor neurons. When a peripheral motor nerve is stimulated at a point proximal to a muscle it activates the muscle to contract. This signal is called the M-wave and can be recorded using EMG electrodes placed on/in that muscle. To obtain maximum activation in the muscle and produce a maximum M-wave (M-max), the amplitude of stimulation is increased until the peak to peak amplitude of the M-wave does not increase further. To ensure maximum simulation, the amplitude of the stimulation is increased by an additional 30%. The amplitude of the M-max is then used to normalize EMG signals from the same muscle during the tasks of interest [97]. Currently, this normalization method is problematic as the repeatability of the M-max is questionable. It seems to be less reliable as the background contraction level increases [98], decreases with time [99], and is dependent on muscle length [100-102] and the task performed [98, 102]. If these factors that affect the M-max values could be controlled resulting in more reliable measurements, this method to normalize EMG data has the potential to facilitate comparisons between muscle, between tasks and between individuals.

4. Summary

In summary, only the normalization method that uses MVICs as the reference level can be validly used to compare muscle activity levels and activation patterns between muscles, tasks and individuals, provided that maximum neural activation is achieved in all muscles and individuals tested. The use of peak or mean activation levels obtained during the task under investigation as the reference EMG level can be used to compare patterns of muscle activation between individuals over time with high reliability but does not allow comparisons of activity levels between muscles, tasks or individuals. The normalization methods of submaximal isometric contractions or maximum activation during the task under investigation performed at maximum effort also do not allow valid comparisons of muscle activity levels between muscles or individuals, and in addition, muscle activation patterns between individuals are potentially more variable because different individual motor control strategies may be used. Finally, the use of maximum activation levels obtained under maximum effort during dynamic contraction and the M-max methods to normalize EMG signals are associated with low within subject reliability and cannot be recommended.

5. EMG Normalization in clinical populations

Studies use EMG to identify differences in the activation levels and patterns between normal subjects and those with neuro-musculo-skeletal dysfunction with the aim of understanding the cause of the dysfunction and developing improved rehabilitation programs to treat the dysfunction. Since the use of MVICs is the most valid method to normalize EMG data allowing comparison of activity levels between muscles in different individuals, it should be the normalization method of choice when evaluating muscle function in clinical populations provided symptomatic individuals can produce MVICs. Indeed recent studies have shown that individuals from some clinical populations (moderate knee osteoarthritis [58], following knee surgery [103], back pain [104, 105], cerebral palsy [106], stroke [45, 107]), are able to produce maximum activation levels using the same MVIC tests as healthy individuals [8]. If symptomatic individuals are unable to elicit maximal contractions, e.g. as a result of pain due to illness or injury, then comparisons between these clinical populations and normal subjects can only be made using normalization to peak or mean activation levels obtained during the task under investigation. Under these circumstances comparisons of activity levels between muscles, between tasks and between individuals are not valid. Only comparison of muscle activation patterns between normal and symptomatic individuals can be made.

Author details

Mark Halaki
Discipline of Exercise and Sport Science, Faculty of Health Science, The University of Sydney, Sydney, Australia

Karen Ginn
Discipline of Biomedical Sciences, Sydney Medical School, The University of Sydney, Sydney, Australia

6. References

[1] Cram JR, Kasman GS. (2011) The basics of surface electromyography. In: Criswell E, Cram JR, editors. Cram's introduction to surface electromyography. 2nd ed. Sudbury, MA: Jones and Bartlett. p. 1-170.

[2]   Basmajian JV (1967) Muscles alive: their functions revealed by electromyography. 2d ed. Baltimore,: Williams & Wilkins; xi, 421 p.

[3]   Cram JR (2003) The history of surface electromyography. Appl Psychophysiol Biofeedback. 28(2):81-91.

[4]   De Luca C (1997) The use of surface electromyography in biomechanics. Journal of Applied Biomechanics. 13:135-63.

[5]   Cram JR, Rommen D (1976) Effects of Skin Preparation on Data Collected Using an EMG Muscle-Scanning Procedure. Biofeedback and Self-Regulation. 14(1).

[6]   Schanne FJ, Chaffin DB (1970) The effects of skin resistance and capacitance coupling on EMG amplitude and power spectra. Electromyography. 10(3):273-86.

[7]   Winkel J, Jorgensen K (1991) Significance of skin temperature changes in surface electromyography. Eur J Appl Physiol Occup Physiol. 63(5):345-8.

[8]   Burden A (2010) How should we normalize electromyograms obtained from healthy participants? What we have learned from over 25 years of research. J Electromyogr Kinesiol. 20(6):1023-35.

[9]   Eberhart HD, Inman VT, Bresler B. (1954) The principal elements in human locomotion. In: Klopsteg PEW, P.D., editor. Human limbs and their substitutes. New York: McGraw-Hill. p. 437-71.

[10] Hodges PW, Richardson CA (1996) Inefficient muscular stabilization of the lumbar spine associated with low back pain. A motor control evaluation of transversus abdominis. Spine (Phila Pa 1976). 21(22):2640-50.

[11] Di Fabio RP (1987) Reliability of computerized surface electromyography for determining the onset of muscle activity. Phys Ther. 67(1):43-8.

[12] Mathiassen SE, Winkel J, Hagg GM (1995) Normalization of surface EMG amplitude from the upper trapezius muscle in ergonomic studies - A review. J Electromyogr Kinesiol. 5(4):197-226.

[13] Erdelyi A, Sihvonen T, Helin P, Hanninen O (1988) Shoulder strain in keyboard workers and its alleviation by arm supports. Int Arch Occup Environ Health. 60(2):119-24.

[14] Granstrom B, Kvarnstrom S, Tiefenbacher F (1985) Electromyography as an aid in the prevention of excessive shoulder strain. Appl Ergon. 16(1):49-54.

[15] Lundervold A (1951) Electromyographic investigations during sedentary work, especially typewriting. Br J Phys Med. 14(2):32-6.

[16] Lundervold AJ (1951) Electromyographic investigations of position and manner of working in typewriting. Acta Physiol Scand Suppl. 24(84):1-171.

[17] Cram JR, Kasman GS, Holtz J (1998) Introduction to surface electromyography. Gaithersburg, Md.: Aspen Publishers; xiv, 408 p.

[18] Perry J (1992) Gait analysis : normal and pathological function. Thorofare, NJ: SLACK; xxxii, 524 p.

[19] Arsenault AB, Winter DA, Marteniuk RG, Hayes KC (1986) How many strides are required for the analysis of electromyographic data in gait? Scand J Rehabil Med. 18(3):133-5.

[20] Neumann DA, Cook TM (1985) Effect of load and carrying position on the electromyographic activity of the gluteus medius muscle during walking. Phys Ther. 65(3):305-11.

[21] Soderberg GL, Cook TM, Rider SC, Stephenitch BL (1991) Electromyographic activity of selected leg musculature in subjects with normal and chronically sprained ankles performing on a BAPS board. Phys Ther. 71(7):514-22.

[22] Woods JJ, Bigland-Ritchie B (1983) Linear and non-linear surface EMG/force relationships in human muscles. An anatomical/functional argument for the existence of both. Am J Phys Med. 62(6):287-99.

[23] Yang JF, Winter DA (1983) Electromyography reliability in maximal and submaximal isometric contractions. Arch Phys Med Rehabil. 64(9):417-20.

[24] Allison GT, Marshall RN, Singer KP (1993) EMG signal amplitude normalization technique in stretch-shortening cycle movements. J Electromyogr Kinesiol. 3(4):236-44.

[25] Yang JF, Winter DA (1984) Electromyographic amplitude normalization methods: improving their sensitivity as diagnostic tools in gait analysis. Arch Phys Med Rehabil. 65(9):517-21.

[26] Allison GT, Godfrey P, Robinson G (1998) EMG signal amplitude assessment during abdominal bracing and hollowing. J Electromyogr Kinesiol. 8(1):51-7.

[27] Ekstrom RA, Soderberg GL, Donatelli RA (2005) Normalization procedures using maximum voluntary isometric contractions for the serratus anterior and trapezius muscles during surface EMG analysis. J Electromyogr Kinesiol. 15(4):418-28.

[28] Gowan ID, Jobe FW, Tibone JE, Perry J, Moynes DR (1987) A comparative electromyographic analysis of the shoulder during pitching. Professional versus amateur pitchers. Am J Sports Med. 15(6):586-90.

[29] Hintermeister RA, Lange GW, Schultheis JM, Bey MJ, Hawkins RJ (1998) Electromyographic activity and applied load during shoulder rehabilitation exercises using elastic resistance. Am J Sports Med. 26(2):210-20.

[30] Harms-Ringdahl K, Ekholm J, Schuldt K, Linder J, Ericson M (1996) Assessment of jet pilots' upper trapezius load calibrated to maximal voluntary contraction and a standardized load. J Electromyogr Kinesiol. 6(1):67-72.

[31] Nordander C, Balogh I, Mathiassen SE, Ohlsson K, Unge J, Skerfving S, et al. (2004) Precision of measurements of physical workload during standardised manual handling. Part I: surface electromyography of m. trapezius, m. infraspinatus and the forearm extensors. J Electromyogr Kinesiol. 14(4):443-54.

[32] Hansson GA, Nordander C, Asterland P, Ohlsson K, Stromberg U, Skerfving S, et al. (2000) Sensitivity of trapezius electromyography to differences between work tasks - influence of gap definition and normalisation methods. J Electromyogr Kinesiol. 10(2):103-15.

[33] Baldisserotto SM, Cosme DC, Loss JF, Shinkai RSA (2010) Reliability of EMG activity in complete denture users during simulation of activities of daily living. Rev odonto ciênc. 25(1):42-7.

[34] Morris AD, Kemp GJ, Lees A, Frostick SP (1998) A study of the reproducibility of three different normalisation methods in intramuscular dual fine wire electromyography of the shoulder. J Electromyogr Kinesiol. 8(5):317-22.

[35] Escamilla RF, McTaggart MS, Fricklas EJ, DeWitt R, Kelleher P, Taylor MK, et al. (2006) An electromyographic analysis of commercial and common abdominal exercises: implications for rehabilitation and training. J Orthop Sports Phys Ther. 36(2):45-57.

[36] Escamilla RF, Lewis C, Bell D, Bramblet G, Daffron J, Lambert S, et al. (2010) Core muscle activation during Swiss ball and traditional abdominal exercises. J Orthop Sports Phys Ther. 40(5):265-76.

[37] Burnett AF, Wee WK, Xie W, Oh PW, Lim JJ, Tan KW (2012) Levels of muscle activation in strength and conditioning exercises and dynamometer hiking in junior sailors. J Strength Cond Res. 26(4):1066-75.

[38] Rouffet DM, Hautier CA (2008) EMG normalization to study muscle activation in cycling. J Electromyogr Kinesiol. 18(5):866-78.

[39] Kankaanpaa M, Taimela S, Laaksonen D, Hanninen O, Airaksinen O (1998) Back and hip extensor fatigability in chronic low back pain patients and controls. Arch Phys Med Rehabil. 79(4):412-7.

[40] Boren K, Conrey C, Le Coguic J, Paprocki L, Voight M, Robinson TK (2011) Electromyographic analysis of gluteus medius and gluteus maximus during rehabilitation exercises. Int J Sports Phys Ther. 6(3):206-23.

[41] Widler KS, Glatthorn JF, Bizzini M, Impellizzeri FM, Munzinger U, Leunig M, et al. (2009) Assessment of hip abductor muscle strength. A validity and reliability study. J Bone Joint Surg Am. 91(11):2666-72.

[42] Bolgla LA, Uhl TL (2007) Reliability of electromyographic normalization methods for evaluating the hip musculature. J Electromyogr Kinesiol. 17(1):102-11.

[43] Purkayastha S, Cramer JT, Trowbridge CA, Fincher AL, Marek SM (2006) Surface electromyographic amplitude-to-work ratios during isokinetic and isotonic muscle actions. J Athl Train. 41(3):314-20.

[44] Albertus-Kajee Y, Tucker R, Derman W, Lamberts RP, Lambert MI (2011) Alternative methods of normalising EMG during running. J Electromyogr Kinesiol. 21(4):579-86.

[45] Hsu WL, Krishnamoorthy V, Scholz JP (2006) An alternative test of electromyographic normalization in patients. Muscle Nerve. 33(2):232-41.

[46] Sousa CO, Ferreira JJA, Veras Medeiros AC, Carvalho AH, Pereira RC, Guedes DT, et al. (2007) Electromyograhic activity in squatting at 40°, 60° and 90° knee flexion positions. Rev Bras Med Esporte. 13(5):280e-6e.

[47] Riemann BL, Limbaugh GK, Eitner JD, LeFavi RG (2011) Medial and lateral gastrocnemius activation differences during heel-raise exercise with three different foot positions. J Strength Cond Res. 25(3):634-9.

[48] Dankaerts W, O'Sullivan PB, Burnett AF, Straker LM, Danneels LA (2004) Reliability of EMG measurements for trunk muscles during maximal and sub-maximal voluntary isometric contractions in healthy controls and CLBP patients. J Electromyogr Kinesiol. 14(3):333-42.

[49] Viitasalo JT, Saukkonen S, Komi PV (1980) Reproducibility of measurements of selected neuromuscular performance variables in man. Electromyogr Clin Neurophysiol. 20(6):487-501.

[50] Winter DA. (1996) EMG interpretation. In: Kumar S, Mital A, editors. Electromyography in ergonomics. London ; Bristol, PA: Taylor & Francis. p. 109-25.

[51] Jobe FW, Moynes DR, Tibone JE, Perry J (1984) An EMG analysis of the shoulder in pitching. A second report. Am J Sports Med. 12(3):218-20.

[52] Chopp JN, Fischer SL, Dickerson CR (2010) On the feasibility of obtaining multiple muscular maximal voluntary excitation levels from test exertions: a shoulder example. J Electromyogr Kinesiol. 20(5):896-902.

[53] Boettcher CE, Ginn KA, Cathers I (2008) Standard maximum isometric voluntary contraction tests for normalizing shoulder muscle EMG. J Orthop Res. 26(12):1591-7.

[54] Kelly BT, Kadrmas WR, Kirkendall DT, Speer KP (1996) Optimal normalization tests for shoulder muscle activation: an electromyographic study. J Orthop Res. 14(4):647-53.

[55] Ekstrom RA, Donatelli RA, Soderberg GL (2003) Surface electromyographic analysis of exercises for the trapezius and serratus anterior muscles. J Orthop Sports Phys Ther. 33(5):247-58.

[56] O'Dwyer NJ, Quinn PT, Guitar BE, Andrews G, Neilson PD (1981) Procedures for verification of electrode placement in EMG studies of orofacial and mandibular muscles. J Speech Hear Res. 24(2):273-88.

[57] Ginn KA, Halaki M, Cathers I (2011) Revision of the Shoulder Normalization Tests is required to include rhomboid major and teres major. J Orthop Res. 29(12):1846-9.

[58] Rutherford DJ, Hubley-Kozey CL, Stanish WD (2011) Maximal voluntary isometric contraction exercises: a methodological investigation in moderate knee osteoarthritis. J Electromyogr Kinesiol. 21(1):154-60.

[59] McGill SM (1991) Electromyographic activity of the abdominal and low back musculature during the generation of isometric and dynamic axial trunk torque: implications for lumbar mechanics. J Orthop Res. 9(1):91-103.

[60] Smith J, Padgett DJ, Kaufman KR, Harrington SP, An KN, Irby SE (2004) Rhomboid muscle electromyography activity during 3 different manual muscle tests. Arch Phys Med Rehabil. 85(6):987-92.

[61] Nieminen H, Takala EP, Viikari-Juntura E (1993) Normalization of electromyogram in the neck-shoulder region. Eur J Appl Physiol Occup Physiol. 67(3):199-207.

[62] Hebert-Losier K, Schneiders AG, Garcia JA, Sullivan SJ, Simoneau GG (2011) Peak triceps surae muscle activity is not specific to knee flexion angles during MVIC. J Electromyogr Kinesiol. 21(5):819-26.

[63] Ekstrom RA, Osborn RW, Goehner HM, Moen AC, Ommen BM, Mefferd MJ, et al. (2012) Electromyographic normalization procedures for determining exercise intensity of closed chain exercises for strengthening the quadriceps femoris muscles. J Strength Cond Res. 26(3):766-71.

[64] Vera-Garcia FJ, Moreside JM, McGill SM (2010) MVC techniques to normalize trunk muscle EMG in healthy women. J Electromyogr Kinesiol. 20(1):10-6.

[65] Ringelberg JA (1985) EMG and force production of some human shoulder muscles during isometric abduction. J Biomech. 18(12):939-47.

[66] Moraes AC, Pinto RS, Valamatos MJ, Pezarat-Correia PL, Okano AH, Santos PM, et al. (2009) EMG activation of abdominal muscles in the crunch exercise performed with different external loads. Phys Ther Sport. 10(2):57-62.

[67] Fernandez-Pena E, Lucertini F, Ditroilo M (2009) A maximal isokinetic pedalling exercise for EMG normalization in cycling. J Electromyogr Kinesiol. 19(3):e162-70.

[68] Liberson WT, Dondey M, Asa MM (1962) Brief repeated isometric maximal exercises. An evaluation by integrative electromyography. Am J Phys Med. 41:3-14.

[69] Inman VT, Ralston HJ, Saunders JB, Feinstein B, Wright EW, Jr. (1952) Relation of human electromyogram to muscular tension. Electroencephalogr Clin Neurophysiol. 4(2):187-94.

[70] Lunnen JD, Yack J, LeVeau BF (1981) Relationship between muscle length, muscle activity, and torque of the hamstring muscles. Phys Ther. 61(2):190-5.

[71] Pincivero DM, Salfetnikov Y, Campy RM, Coelho AJ (2004) Angle- and gender-specific quadriceps femoris muscle recruitment and knee extensor torque. J Biomech. 37(11):1689-97.

[72] Kasprisin JE, Grabiner MD (1998) EMG variability during maximum voluntary isometric and anisometric contractions is reduced using spatial averaging. J Electromyogr Kinesiol. 8(1):45-50.

[73] Leedham JS, Dowling JJ (1995) Force-length, torque-angle and EMG-joint angle relationships of the human in vivo biceps brachii. Eur J Appl Physiol Occup Physiol. 70(5):421-6.

[74] Barr AE, Goldsheyder D, Ozkaya N, Nordin M (2001) Testing apparatus and experimental procedure for position specific normalization of electromyographic measurements of distal upper extremity musculature. Clin Biomech (Bristol, Avon). 16(7):576-85.

[75] Mohamed O, Perry J, Hislop H (2002) Relationship between wire EMG activity, muscle length, and torque of the hamstrings. Clin Biomech (Bristol, Avon). 17(8):569-79.

[76] Okada M (1987) Effect of muscle length on surface EMG wave forms in isometric contractions. Eur J Appl Physiol Occup Physiol. 56(4):482-6.

[77] Mirka GA (1991) The quantification of EMG normalization error. Ergonomics. 34(3):343-52.

[78] Burden AM, Trew M, Baltzopoulos V (2003) Normalisation of gait EMGs: a re-examination. J Electromyogr Kinesiol. 13(6):519-32.

[79] Heckathorne CW, Childress DS (1981) Relationships of the surface electromyogram to the force, length, velocity, and contraction rate of the cineplastic human biceps. Am J Phys Med. 60(1):1-19.

[80] Hales JP, Gandevia SC (1988) Assessment of maximal voluntary contraction with twitch interpolation: an instrument to measure twitch responses. J Neurosci Methods. 25(2):97-102.

[81] Gandevia SC, McKenzie DK (1985) Activation of the human diaphragm during maximal static efforts. J Physiol. 367:45-56.

[82] Gandevia SC, McKenzie DK (1988) Activation of human muscles at short muscle lengths during maximal static efforts. J Physiol. 407:599-613.

[83] Merton PA (1954) Voluntary strength and fatigue. J Physiol. 123(3):553-64.

[84] Belanger AY, McComas AJ (1981) Extent of motor unit activation during effort. J Appl Physiol. 51(5):1131-5.

[85] Bigland-Ritchie B, Woods JJ (1984) Changes in muscle contractile properties and neural control during human muscular fatigue. Muscle Nerve. 7(9):691-9.

[86] Winter DA, Yack HJ (1987) EMG profiles during normal human walking: stride-to-stride and inter-subject variability. Electroencephalogr Clin Neurophysiol. 67(5):402-11.

[87] Chapman AR, Vicenzino B, Blanch P, Knox JJ, Hodges PW (2010) Intramuscular fine-wire electromyography during cycling: repeatability, normalisation and a comparison to surface electromyography. J Electromyogr Kinesiol. 20(1):108-17.

[88] Trevithick BA, Ginn KA, Halaki M, Balnave R (2007) Shoulder muscle recruitment patterns during a kayak stroke performed on a paddling ergometer. J Electromyogr Kinesiol. 17(1):74-9.

[89] Burden A, Bartlett R (1999) Normalisation of EMG amplitude: an evaluation and comparison of old and new methods. Med Eng Phys. 21(4):247-57.

[90] Knutson LM, Soderberg GL, Ballantyne BT, Clarke WR (1994) A study of various normalization procedures for within day electromyographic data. J Electromyogr Kinesiol. 4(1):47-59.

[91] Veiersted KB (1991) The reproducibility of test contractions for calibration of electromyographic measurements. Eur J Appl Physiol Occup Physiol. 62(2):91-8.

[92] Bao S, Mathiassen SE, Winkel J (1995) Normalizing upper trapezius EMG amplitude: Comparison of different procedures. J Electromyogr Kinesiol. 5(4):251-7.

[93] Lehman GJ (2002) Clinical considerations in the use of surface electromyography: three experimental studies. J Manipulative Physiol Ther. 25(5):293-9.

[94] Mathiassen SE, Winkel J (1990) Electromyographic activity in the shoulder-neck region according to arm position and glenohumeral torque. Eur J Appl Physiol Occup Physiol. 61(5-6):370-9.

[95] Ounpuu S, Winter DA (1989) Bilateral electromyographical analysis of the lower limbs during walking in normal adults. Electroencephalogr Clin Neurophysiol. 72(5):429-38.

[96] Anders C, Bretschneider S, Bernsdorf A, Schneider W (2005) Activation characteristics of shoulder muscles during maximal and submaximal efforts. Eur J Appl Physiol. 93(5-6):540-6.

[97] Pucci AR, Griffin L, Cafarelli E (2006) Maximal motor unit firing rates during isometric resistance training in men. Exp Physiol. 91(1):171-8.

[98] Lee M, Carroll TJ (2005) The amplitude of Mmax in human wrist flexors varies during different muscle contractions despite constant posture. J Neurosci Methods. 149(2):95-100.

[99] Crone C, Johnsen LL, Hultborn H, Orsnes GB (1999) Amplitude of the maximum motor response (Mmax) in human muscles typically decreases during the course of an experiment. Exp Brain Res. 124(2):265-70.

[100] Maffiuletti NA, Lepers R (2003) Quadriceps femoris torque and EMG activity in seated versus supine position. Med Sci Sports Exerc. 35(9):1511-6.

[101] Cresswell AG, Loscher WN, Thorstensson A (1995) Influence of gastrocnemius muscle length on triceps surae torque development and electromyographic activity in man. Exp Brain Res. 105(2):283-90.

[102] Tucker KJ, Tuncer M, Turker KS (2005) A review of the H-reflex and M-wave in the human triceps surae. Hum Mov Sci. 24(5-6):667-88.

[103] Krebs DE (1989) Isokinetic, electrophysiologic, and clinical function relationships following tourniquet-aided knee arthrotomy. Phys Ther. 69(10):803-15.

[104] Ng JK, Richardson CA, Parnianpour M, Kippers V (2002) Fatigue-related changes in torque output and electromyographic parameters of trunk muscles during isometric axial rotation exertion: an investigation in patients with back pain and in healthy subjects. Spine (Phila Pa 1976). 27(6):637-46.

[105] Ng JK, Richardson CA, Parnianpour M, Kippers V (2002) EMG activity of trunk muscles and torque output during isometric axial rotation exertion: a comparison between back pain patients and matched controls. J Orthop Res. 20(1):112-21.

[106] Damiano DL, Martellotta TL, Sullivan DJ, Granata KP, Abel MF (2000) Muscle force production and functional performance in spastic cerebral palsy: relationship of cocontraction. Arch Phys Med Rehabil. 81(7):895-900.

[107] Mulroy S, Gronley J, Weiss W, Newsam C, Perry J (2003) Use of cluster analysis for gait pattern classification of patients in the early and late recovery phases following stroke. Gait Posture. 18(1):114-25.

Chapter 2

Nonlinear Analysis of Surface EMG Signals

Min Lei and Guang Meng

Additional information is available at the end of the chapter

1. Introduction

The aim of this chapter is to answer the essence of SEMG and to explore the potential use of nonlinear analysis as a tool in the clinical and biomechanical applications. The technical tools include nonlinear time series test, time series analysis based on chaos theory, multifractal analysis.

In Section 2, we discuss the two methods of nonlinear time series test: surrogate data test method and Volterra-Wiener-Korenberg (VWK) model test method. Theoretically, the two methods can detect the nonlinearity of the data indirectly. The surrogate data method is used to analyze the SEMG. The result shows that the SEMG has deterministic nonlinear components. Meanwhile, we introduce the VWK model test method and compare it with the surrogate data method. The nonlinearity of SEMG during muscle fatigue can be detected by the VWK.

In Section 3, we describe the time series analysis based on chaos theory. The chaos definition and chaotic characteristics are discussed. The embedding theory of the attractor reconstruction is investigated for the dynamical system. From the view of the fractal structure of the chaotic attractor, the correlation dimension is used to test the chaotic characteristics of the SEMG during arm movements. The Largest Lyapunov exponent is also studied. Then, we investigate the influence of measure noise, internal noise and sampling interval on the principal components of chaotic time series. The symplectic principal component analysis is given. We illustrate the feasibility of this method and give the embedding dimension of the action surface EMG signal.

In Section 4, the self-affine fractal definition and nature are described. The power spectrum and frequency relationship is used to calculate the self-affine fractal dimension of the time series, such as SEMG. Then, the multifractal dimension is given for the SEMG.

The conclusion and future research are shown in Section 5. Here, it is necessary to note that this chapter is actually the result of many years work. The new methods presented here build on a broad and strong foundation of nonlinear time series analysis and chaotic dynamical theory.

2. Detecting nonlinearity of the surface EMG signals

In many areas of science and engineering, it is a critical issue to determine whether an observed time series is purely stochastic, or deterministic nonlinear, even chaotic. One may know about the intrinsic properties of the observed phenomenon by distinguishing between nonlinear deterministic dynamics and noisy dynamics from a time series. In this section, we review and discuss the surrogate data test method[1] and Volterra-Wiener-Korenberg (VWK) model test method[2] for identifying the nonlinearity of a time series. These methods have been successfully used to detect and characterize nonlinear dynamics from recordings in biology and medicine[2-5].

Surrogate analysis is currently an important empirical technique of testing nonlinearity for a time series. The aim is to test whether the dynamics are consistent with linearly filtered noise or a nonlinear dynamical system[1, 6]. The basic idea of the surrogate data method is to first specify some kind of linear stochastic process as a null hypothesis that mimics "linear properties" of the original data. According to the null hypothesis, surrogate data sets are generated. Then, a discriminating statistic is calculated for the original and for each of the surrogate data sets. If the statistic of the original data is significantly different from those of surrogate data sets, the null hypothesis can be rejected within a certain confidence level. It shows that the original data is from a nonlinear dynamical system. The method is demonstrated for numerical time series generated by known chaotic systems and applied to the analysis of SEMG.

VWK test method is a kind of nonlinear detection of time series based on linear and nonlinear Volterra-Wiener-Korenberg model [2, 5]. That is, it first produces the linear and nonlinear predicted data from the original time series and then compares their information criterions to detect the nonlinearity of the raw data. VWK test technique is capable of robust and highly sensitive statistical detection of deterministic dynamics, including chaotic dynamics, in experimental time series. This method is superior to other techniques when applied to short time series, either continuous or discrete, even when heavily contaminated with noise or in the presence of strong periodicity. Later, an extension of the Volterra algorithm (called the numerical titration algorithm) was given to detect and quantify chaos in noisy time series[7]. Here, the surrogate data method and VWK test approach are used to analyze the nonlinearity of surface EMG signals.

2.1. Surrogate data test method

Surrogate data method includes two parts: a null hypothesis and a test statistic. The null hypothesis is a specific process which may or may not adequately explain an origin of the data. The test statistic provides a quantitative description to demonstrate the data sources.

2.1.1. Null hypotheses and algorithms[1]

The null hypotheses usually specify some certain properties of the original data that reflect some structure characteristics of the dynamical system, such as mean and variance, and possibly also the Fourier power spectrum. Different null hypotheses describe different specific dynamical systems. In terms of the corresponding null hypothesis, the surrogate data can be generated so as to test the corresponding specific dynamical system class.

Null hypothesis 1 The observed data is produced by independent and identically distributed (IID) random variables.

For this hypothesis, the corresponding surrogate data can be generated by shuffling the time-order of the original time series so that it has the same mean, variance and amplitude distribution as the original data. But any temporal correlations of the original data are destroyed in the surrogate data. Schienkman and LeBaron[8] applied this hypothesis to analyze stock market returns. Breeden and Packard also used this hypothesis to demonstrate that a time series of quasar data which were sampled nonuniformly in time has some dynamics structure[9].

The algorithm of the null hypothesis is that one first create gaussian random numbers from 1 to N, where N is the length of the original data x. Then, the original data x is permuted by the random numbers to generate the surrogate data.

Null hypothesis 2 The observed data is produced by the Ornstein-Uhlenbeck process.

The surrogate data generated by the Ornstein-Uhlenbeck process is a sequence that has the simplest time correlation. The Ornstein-Uhlenbeck process can be given as follows.

$$x_t = a_0 + a_1 x_{t-1} + \sigma e_t \tag{1}$$

where e_t is a Gaussian random with zero mean and unit variance. The coefficients a_0, a_1, and σ work together to determine the mean, variance, and autocorrelation time of the time series x_t. In this case, its autocorrelation function is exponential form. Let $\lambda = -\log a_1$, $\langle \cdot \rangle$ denotes an average over time t. That is,

$$A(\tau) \equiv \frac{\langle x_t \cdot x_{t-\tau} \rangle - \langle x_t \rangle^2}{\langle x_t^2 \rangle - \langle x_t \rangle^2} = e^{-\lambda|\tau|} \tag{2}$$

In order to generate the surrogate data that is consistent with this hypothesis, the algorithm is that one first calculates the mean μ, variance γ and autocorrelation $A(1)$ (in Eq. (2)) from the original data x. Then, the coefficients in Eq. (1) can be estimated: $a_1 = A(1)$, $a_0 = \mu(1-a_1)$, and $\sigma^2 = \gamma(1-a_1^2)$. The Gaussian e_t can be generated by a pseudorandom number generator. Finally, the surrogate data can be produced by iterating Eq. (1).

Null hypothesis 3 The observed data is produced by the linear autocorrelated gaussian process with the mean and variance of the original time series.

The hypothesis has been usually used to test whether the original time series contains nonlinear components. It can be described by using a linear autoregressive (AR) model.

$$x_t = a_0 + \sum_{k=1}^{q} a_k x_{t-k} + \sigma e_t \tag{3}$$

There are the two algorithms to produce the surrogate data in accord with this hypothesis. One algorithm is to directly use Eq.3. That is, the coefficients are firstly identified by using the original data. Then, the surrogate data is generated by repeatedly iterating Eq.3. However, the performance of this algorithm is very unstable. If the values of the coefficients are mis-estimated slightly, this algorithm may lead to the iterative results which easily diverge to infinity. The alternative algorithm is that a surrogate data is generated by randomizing the phases of a Fourier transform. According to the Weiner-Khintchine theorem, the two algorithms are equivalent in essence[1, 10]. The surrogate data has the same Fourier spectrum as the original data. Meanwhile, the algorithm based on the Fourier transform is stabler in the numerical calculation than the first algorithm. The following is the steps of this algorithm.

Let an observed data as $x(n)$. The Fourier transform of $x(n)$ is computed as follows[3]:

$$X(k) = \sum_{n=0}^{N-1} x(n)e^{-2\pi i n k / N} \tag{4}$$

The Fourier transform has a complex amplitude at each frequency. One can randomize the phases of the Fourier transform by multiplying $e^{i\varphi}$,

$$X'(k) = X(k) \cdot e^{i\varphi} \tag{5}$$

where φ is independently chosen for each frequency from the $[0, 2\pi]$. In order to the inverse Fourier transform to be real (no imaginary components), the phases must satisfy the antisymmetric condition $\varphi(k) = -\varphi(N-k)$. Meanwhile, $\varphi(0) = 0$, $\varphi(N/2) = 0$ (when N is even), so that

$$X'(k) = \overline{X'(N-k)} \tag{6}$$

This point can be easily proved[11].

Proof:

According to the nature of DFT of a real time series $x(n)$, if $x(n) \in R$, then

$$\phi(k) = -\phi(-k) \tag{7}$$

where $\phi(k)$ is the phase angle of $X(k)$. $k = 0, 1, \ldots$ N-1. N is the period of Fourier Transform. Then, for $k = 0$, $k = N/2$ (N is even), there are

$$\phi(0) = -\phi(0), \tag{8}$$

$$\phi(N/2) = -\phi(-N/2) = -\phi(N/2) \tag{9}$$

In order to ensure that the inverse Fourier transform results are real values, there must be

$$\phi(0) = 0 \,, \quad \phi(N/2) = 0 \,.$$

In practical, if the data length N is odd, $\varphi(f_1)=0$, $\varphi(f_i) = -\varphi(f_k)$, $i=2\sim(N+1)/2$, $k=N\sim(N+1)/2+1$; If N is even, $\varphi(f_1)=0$, $\varphi(f_{N/2+1})=0$, $\varphi(f_i)=-\varphi(f_k)$, $i=2\sim N/2$, $k=N\sim N/2+2$. Thus, the surrogate data $x'(n)$ given by the inverse Fourier transform is a sequence of real numbers.

$$x'(n) = \frac{1}{N} \sum_{k=0}^{N-1} X'(k) \cdot e^{2\pi i n k / N} \tag{10}$$

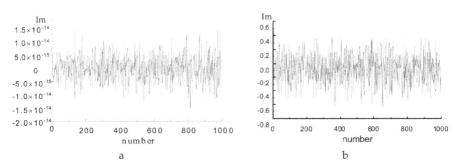

Figure 1. The imaginary components of surrogate data by our (a) and previous (b) FT algorithm

Thus, there are no imaginary components (see Fig. (1a)). The values of the imaginary parts are very little (magnitude 10^{-14}) so that they can be regarded as computing precision errors. The surrogate data has the same Fourier transform spectrum as the original data by using this algorithm. The reproduced "pure" frequencies are very well. Fig.(1b)shows that the previous FT algorithm[1] cannot make the imaginary components of Fourier inverse transform to be zero. So, if one only uses the real part of Fourier inverse transform as surrogate data and omit its imaginary components, the obtained surrogates would have the two limitations[1, 12].

Null hypothesis 4 The observed data is produced by the static nonlinear transform of linear gaussian process.

The static nonlinear transform is that the observation or measure function is nonlinear. The static means that the measure data x_t only depends on the state y_t of the dynamic process at the time t, not on derivatives or values in the past. Let h be a measure function, then

$$x_t = h(y_t) \tag{11}$$

The generated surrogate data not only contain the linear correlated characteristic, but also can reflect the static, monotonic nonlinearity of the original data. Strictly speaking, time series in this class are nonlinear. But this nonlinearity is not from the dynamics. This hypothesis can be used to indicate whether the nonlinearity is from the dynamical system or the amplitude distribution (i.e. the measure process).

For generating surrogate data corresponding to this null hypothesis, an algorithm is described. The aim is to shuffle the time-order of the data x_t and to preserve the linear correlations of the underlying time series $y_t = h^{-1}(x_t)$. The first step is to make a Gaussian time series y_t, where each element is generated independently from a Gaussian pseudorandom number generator. Next, we rescale y_t in accordance with the time-order of the original data x_t. The re-ordered y_t has a time series which "follows" the static, monotonic nonlinearity of the original data. Then, the data y'_t is created by using the above FT algorithm to deal with the re-ordered y_t. Finally, the raw data x_t is rescaled in terms of the time-order of the data y'_t to generate the surrogate data x'_t. The "underlying" time series (y_t and y'_t) are Gaussian and have the same Fourier power spectrum. The produced x'_t matches the amplitude distribution of the raw data x_t.

2.1.2. Test statistics[6]

The test statistic is a value which estimates some certain aspects of the time series. To compare the raw data to its surrogate data sets, a suitable test statistic must be selected. A useful statistic should be pivotal and independent of the way that surrogate data sets are generated. In other words, for every data set z and every realization z_i of any $F_i \in F_{\phi}$, their test statistics should be different, i.e.

$$T(z) \neq T(z_i) \tag{12}$$

where F_{ϕ} represents the null hypothesis process. Meanwhile, the distribution of T under the null hypothesis does not depend on μ or σ. Here we give two discriminating statistics as follows:

$$T = \overline{(x - \bar{x})^4} \Big/ \overline{(x - \bar{x})^2}^2 \tag{13}$$

$$T = \frac{1}{n-1} \sum_{i=1}^{n-1} \left| (x(i) - \bar{x}) \cdot (x(i+1) - \bar{x}) \right| \Big/ \overline{(x - \bar{x})^2} \tag{14}$$

where "$\bar{\ }$" denotes the average of the data. The mean μ and variance σ have no effect on the T value in Eq. (13). Therefore, some linear structure characteristics can be determined except for the mean and variance. The T value in Eq.(14) can judge if the surrogate data are consist with the raw data in the view of the correlation with the mean and variance. The T value in Eq. (15) is a simple skewed difference statistic that is both rapidly computable and often quite powerful.

$$T = \left\langle (x_{t+m} - x_t)^3 \right\rangle \Big/ \left\langle (x_{t+m} - x_t)^2 \right\rangle \tag{15}$$

where $\langle \cdot \rangle$ is mean operator, m is time delay. This statistic T provides a more significant rejection of the hypothesis of the static nonlinear filter of an underlying linear process. Informally, this statistic indicates the asymmetry between rise and fall times in the time series.

2.1.3. Performance of surrogate data method based on our FT algorithm[3, 13, 14]

The surrogate data method is suitable to detect the nonlinearity of a short, noisy time series. Here, a Gaussian data and a Logistic chaotic time series are used to study the performance of surrogate data method. For a two-sided test, the probability of rejecting the null hypothesis is given by the confidence level p, the surrogate data sets B must be at least as large as $B_{min} = 2/(1 - p) - 1$. For 95% confidence level, there should be 39 sets of surrogate data.

A Gaussian data x is a random time series with zero mean and unit variance produced by the pseudorandom generator. The data length is 1000 points. According to the null hypothesis 3, 39 sets of surrogate data are generated by using our above FT algorithm. The T value is calculated by Eq. (13) and Eq. (14), respectively. In the Figure (2a and b), there are no statistical discrepancy between the test statistic T of the raw data x and those of surrogate data.

The statistic T values of the raw data are on the range of the empirical distribution of T given by the surrogate data. The results show that the generated surrogate data has the same Fourier transform spectrum as the raw data besides the same mean and variance as the raw data because the T value in Eq. (14) is a measure of the time irreversibility of the data. The null hypothesis 3 is accepted at the confidence level 95%. The raw data is consistent with the stochastic process of the null hypothesis 3. The surrogate data produced by the above FT algorithm is equivalent to the raw data. The generated surrogate data reflects the null hypothesis 3.

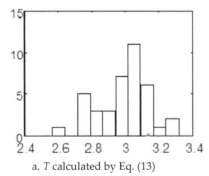 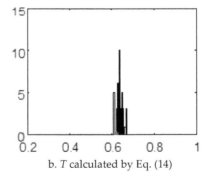

a. T calculated by Eq. (13)   b. T calculated by Eq. (14)

Figure 2. The histogram is T distribution of surrogate data given by FT algorithm, * is T value of the original data, where abscissa is T, ordinate is the number of surrogate data sets

To further test that the surrogate data based on the above FT algorithm can be used to detect nonlinearity of a time series, we apply the Logistic chaotic system to produce a chaotic time series as follows.

$$x_{t+1} = \alpha x_t (1 - x_t) + e \qquad (16)$$

where $\alpha = 3.9$, $x_0 \in [0,1]$, e is white noise with mean 0, variance 0.001^2. If e takes part in the evolution process of the above equation, it is called as interior noise (or dynamic noise); otherwise it is called as measure noise.

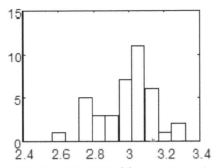 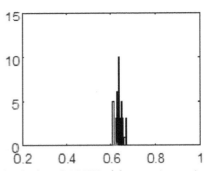

a. The length N=5000 of the raw time series   b. The length N=500 of the raw time series

Figure 3. T calculated by Eq. (13), histogram is T distribution of surrogate data, * is T value of the original data, where abscissa is T, ordinate is the number of surrogate data sets

For the case without noise $e = 0$, we use Eq. (16) to compute the two Logistic chaotic time series with the length of 5000 points and 500 points. 39 surrogate data generated by the above FT algorithm contain the linear properties of the original data in terms of the null hypothesis 3. In Fig.3, we can see the obvious difference between the original data and its surrogate data, regardless of the length of 5000 points or 500 points. The null hypothesis can be rejected in 95% confidence level. The original data has nonlinear components. The results show that the data length has little effect on the surrogate data method based on the above FT algorithm. In Figure 4, we study the nonlinear test of Logistic chaotic time series with measure noise and interior noise, respectively. The data length is 1000 points. According to the null hypothesis, 39 sets of surrogate data are generated. The statistic T for the original data is significantly different from the values obtained for the surrogate data sets. The null hypothesis 3 can also be rejected in 95% significance. The nonlinearity of the original data can be detected. To sum up, the length and noise has no impact on the surrogate data method based on our FT algorithm.

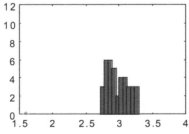 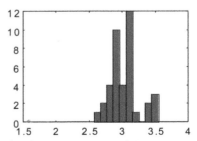

a. Chaos time series with measure noise   b. Chaos time series with interior noise

Figure 4. T calculated by Eq.(13), histogram is T distribution of surrogate data, * is T value of the original data, where abscissa is T, ordinate is the number of surrogate data sets

2.1.4. Nonlinear test of surface EMG signal based on surrogate data[3, 13, 14]

The nature of SEMG plays an important role in neuromuscular disorder diagnosis, muscle fatigue monitoring, prosthesis control, etc. Here the analyzed data are collected from physiological instruments. Humid surface electrode and AD12-16LG collecting card of physiology signal are used in the whole experiment that was done at Hua Shan Hospital in Shanghai. The data are sampled at 1kHz for the action surface EMG (ASEMG) [3]and the fatigue surface EMG (FSEMG) when one hand carries a 1kg heavy thing [15](see Fig. 5). The length of data for ASEMG is 1000 points during the beginning of action because this time span contains the information of the forearm movement. In the case of carrying a 1kg heavy thing, the length of FSEMG data is also 1000 points when the arm has been fatigue.

For these surface EMG signals, 39 surrogate data are produced by the null hypothesis 2. The surrogate data analysis is given for the action surface EMG signal and the fatigue surface EMG signal, respectively(see Fig. 6). The results show that for action surface EMG signal and fatigue surface EMG signal, their T values are obviously different from those of surrogate data in terms of Eq.13. The null hypothesis 2 can be rejected in 95% degree of confidence. The action surface EMG signal and fatigue surface EMG signal is not stochastic signal produced by a linear stochastic process, but contains nonlinear components. However, this result could not ensure that this nonlinearity must be from the dynamic system.

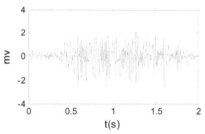
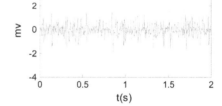

a. a typical action surface EMG wave   b. a typical fatigue surface EMG wave

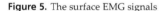

Figure 5. The surface EMG signals

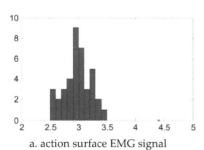
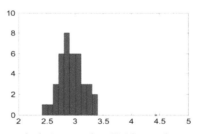

a. action surface EMG signal   b. fatigue surface EMG signal

Figure 6. Surrogate data analysis of surface EMG signal. * is T_{orig}, histogram is T_{surr} distribution of surrogate data

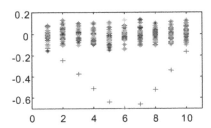

Figure 7. Surrogate data test of surface EMG signal during movement, where surrogate data sets are 39 sets; * is T value of surrogate data by the null hypothesis 4, +is T value of EMG signal, where T is calculated by Eq. 15

In order to test that the nonlinear components are intrinsic deterministic, we further assume that ASEMG is stochastic signal consistent with the null hypothesis 4. Fig.7 gives the T values of ASEMG and surrogate data calculated by Eq. 15. This statistic indicates the asymmetry between rise and fall times in the time series. From this figure, we can see that there is the difference between data and surrogates, and the null hypothesis 4 is rejected in 95% credibility. This result shows that the nonlinearity of ASEMG is intrinsic and deterministic.

2.2. Volterra-Wiener-Korenberg test method

2.2.1. Volterra-Wiener-Korenberg test model[2]

For a dynamic system, an observed time series $\{y_n\}_{n=1}^N$ can be treated as a closed loop Volterra series by utilizing the feedback of y_n. Suppose the time series is univariate. A discrete Volterra-Winner-Korenberg series can be calculated as follows:

$$
\begin{aligned}
y_n^{cala} &= a_0 + a_1 y_{n-1} + a_2 y_{n-2} + \cdots + a_k y_{n-k} + a_{k+1} y_{n-1}^2 + a_{k+2} y_{n-1} y_{n-2} + \cdots + a_{M-1} y_{n-k}^d \\
&= \sum_{m=0}^{M} a_m z_m(n)
\end{aligned}
\tag{17}
$$

where the memory k and combination degree d correspond to the embedding dimension and the degree of nonlinearity of the model, respectively. The coefficients a_m are recursively estimated through a Gram-Schmidt procedure from linear and nonlinear autocorrelations of the data itself with a total dimension $M=(k+d)!/(d!k!)$.

There is the following information criterion in accordance with the parsimony principle:

$$
C(r) = \log \varepsilon(r) + r/N
\tag{18}
$$

$$
\varepsilon(k,d)^2 \equiv \frac{\sum_{n=1}^{N} (y_a^{calc}(k,d) - y_n)^2}{\sum_{n=1}^{N} (y_n - \bar{y})^2}
\tag{19}
$$

where $r \in [1, M]$ is the number of polynomial terms of the truncated Volterra expansions from the given pair $\{k, d\}$, $\varepsilon(k,d)^2$ is a normalized variance of the error residuals, $\bar{y} = \frac{1}{N}\sum_{n=1}^{N} y_n$. For $d=1$, VWK model is linear, whereas the model is nonlinear for $d>1$.

For each data series, there is the following numerical procedure to search for the optimal pair $\{k_{opt}, d_{opt}\}$:

1. when $d=1$, search for k_{opt} which minimizes $C(r)$.
2. with $k=k_{opt}$, increasing $d>1$, search for d_{opt} which minimizes $C(r)$.
3. calculate $C^{lin}(r)$ with $d=1$ and $k=M-1$, and $C^{nl}(r)$ with $d=d_{opt}$ and $k=k_{opt}$.
4. Compare $C^{lin}(r)$ and $C^{nl}(r)$, if $C^{nl}(r)$ is obviously smaller than $C^{lin}(r)$, then the original system dynamics is nonlinear, the obtained time series is nonlinear, even chaos; otherwise, the original system dynamics is linear, the raw data is linear.

Note that when k_{opt} is rather large, M is quite large, too, then the computational time will rapidly go up. In this case, k and d should be adjusted synchronously to search for k_{opt} and d_{opt} so as to make $C^{nl}(r) < C^{lin}(r)$. Furthermore, one can obtain the corresponding linear and nonlinear models for surrogate data generated by the FT algorithm according to the null hypothesis 3 so that $C^{lin}_{orig}(r)$, $C^{lin}_{surr}(r)$, $C^{nl}_{surr}(r) > C^{nl}_{orig}(r)$ in the statistical sense.

2.2.2. Analysis of SEMG based on VWK method[15, 16]

Here, the VWK method is used to deal with the surface EMG signals in Fig.5. For the action surface EMG signal, $C^{lin}(r)$ is almost equal to $C^{nl}(r)$, i.e. $C^{lin}(r) \approx C^{nl}(r)$, this technique can hardly detect its nonlinearity (see Fig.8a). For the fatigue surface EMG signal, $C^{nl}(r)$ is distinctly smaller than $C^{lin}(r)$ so that its nonlinear component can be detected (see Fig.8b). So VWK technique can effectively detect the nonlinear dynamic speciality of fatigue surface EMG signal but fails to test the nonlinearity of the action surface EMG signal. In other words, VWK technique can not be used directly to deal with the action surface EMG signal.

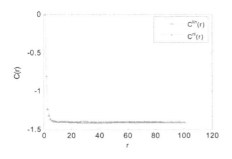
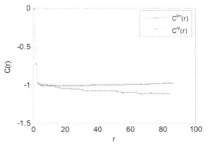

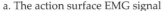

a. The action surface EMG signal   b. The fatigue surface EMG signal

Figure 8. VWK test analysis of surface EMG signal

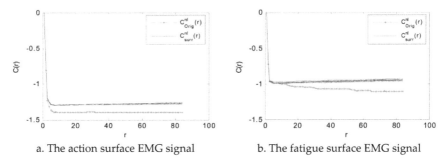

a. The action surface EMG signal   b. The fatigue surface EMG signal

Figure 9. VWK combined with surrogate analysis of surface EMG signal. solid is $C_{surr}^{nl}(r)$, * is $C_{orig}^{nl}(r)$

2.2.3. Analysis of SEMG based on VWK method with surrogate data[16]

In order to detect the nonlinearity of the action surface EMG signal, 39 FT-based surrogate data are used according to the null hypothesis 3. The generated surrogate data contain the linear properties of the raw data. Figure 9 is the analysis of surface EMG signal based on VWK with surrogate data. We can see that no matter whether it is the action or fatigue EMG signal, $C_{orig}^{nl}(r)$ is always smaller than $C_{surr}^{nl}(r)$. The null hypothesis 3 can be rejected in 95% significance. The results illuminate that the action and fatigue surface EMG signals contain nonlinear dynamic properties.

3. Analysis of the surface EMG signals based on chaos theory

The discovery of chaotic phenomena is the third major breakthrough in the 20th century physics scientific community following the creation of relativity and quantum mechanics. It organically combines the two major theoretical systems of determinism and probabilism that have long been debated to create a scientific model of a new paradigm, so that people can use some simple rules to explain seemingly stochastic information in the past[17-19]. The practical significance that finds chaotic phenomena is to recognize that a deterministic nonlinear system can have inherent uncertainty. Perhaps a system has only a few degrees of freedom, but it can produce complex, similar to the random output signal. In the past, one could only denote a random-looking data as a random process from the view of the traditional time series analysis. The statistical methods or random time series models were used to analyze the data. Since the chaotic phenomenon was discovered by Lorenz[17], people have begun to reunderstand and restudy these random-looking signals so as to reveal the inherent deterministic mechanisms of these signals. That is, it is to explore that the systems which generate these signals may contain essentially deterministic characteristics. Chaos phenomenon breaks the path that the regularity is found in a lot of completely different systems. This will lead to a revolution in the field of influence of various disciplines. It is chaos to lead people to explore the complexity in nature.

At present, the idea of Chaos has been introduced into the analysis of time series to create the field of chaotic time series analysis. Since the inception of chaotic time series analysis, it has quickly been penetrated into other disciplines and engineering fields. Thus it becomes the most active branch of the modern nonlinear dynamics. This section describes the chaos definition and the phase space reconstruction of chaotic time series, discusses some parameters that are used to analysis chaotic time series, such as the correlation dimension and Lyapunov exponent, study the principal component analysis methods based on SVD, and propose the symplectic principal component method based on symplectic geometry. Then we use these methods to investigate the surface EMG signals.

3.1. Chaos and its definition

Chaos is "order in disorder". The order means its deterministic nature. The disorder means that the final results can be unpredictable for a long time. As a scientific concept, chaos generally denotes that the long-term dynamical behavior of a deterministic nonlinear system manifests as a random-looking behavior. Mathematically speaking, "chaos" has not been a unified strict definition. For the definition of chaos, there are at least nine different definitions, where the three definitions given by Li-Yorke, Devaney, Marotto are more commonly used. Here describes the definition of chaos by Li-Yorke[18].

Li-Yorke Theorem: Let $f(x)$ as a continuous self-map in $[a, b]$. If $f(x)$ has a periodic point with period 3, then for any positive integer $n=1, 2, 3, \ldots$, there is a periodic point with period n.

This is the famous period 3 theorem. It becomes a milestone in the development history of chaos theory and promotes the creation and development of chaos theory. From this theorem, the first formal mathematical definition of the chaos is given.

Chaos definition: Let $f(x)$ as a continuous self-map in closed interval I, i.e.

$$f : I \to I \subset R^m, \quad y = f(x) \tag{20}$$

where $x, y \in I$. If $m = 1$, f is one-dimensional mapping. If $m \neq 1$, f is multi-dimensional mapping. Denote the n times iteration of f as $f^n(x)$. If Eq.20 satisfies the following conditions, then it has chaotic motion:

1. The period of periodic point of f has no upper bound.
2. There is an uncountable set $S \subset I$, which satisfies the following conditions:

$$\lim_{n \to \infty} \sup \left| f^n(x) - f^n(y) \right| > 0, \qquad \forall x, y \in S, \quad x \neq y \tag{21}$$

$$\lim_{n \to \infty} \inf \left| f^n(x) - f^n(y) \right| = 0, \qquad \forall x, y \in S \tag{22}$$

$$\lim_{n \to \infty} \sup \left| f^n(x) - f^n(p) \right| > 0, \qquad \forall x \in S, \quad \forall p \in P(f) \tag{23}$$

where $P(f) \underline{\underline{\Delta}} \{x \mid x$ is a periodic point of $f\}$.

This definition explains "existence" of chaos in mathematics. According to the above theorem and the definition, the description of chaotic motion is different from the general periodic and quasi-periodic motion. Its motion is not a single periodic orbit but an envelope for a bunch of tracks, where the infinite number of countable stable periodic orbits and uncountable stable aperiodic orbits are embedded densely. Meanwhile, there is at least one unstable aperiodic orbit. Overall, the chaos not only contains some inherent regularity, but also shows that the system has ergodicity. That is, the system has a long-term unpredictability. In other words, the long-term behavior of the system can not be predicted if the system displays the so-called "sensitive dependence on initial conditions". The meaning of this definition is that the aperiodicity of chaotic system is exhibited accurately. For a dynamical system, the observable behaviour was called stochastic in the past. In fact, it can be random-looking, i.e. "stochastic behaviour occurring in a deterministic system". Therefore, it is challenging to quantitatively describe the nature of chaotic dynamics and distinguish between the so-called random and chaotic motions from a time series, especially from an experimental time series. At present, chaotic time series analysis methods have been widely attention in fields of mathematics, physics, biology, biomedicine, robotics, geology, engineering, economics, finance, and so on.

3.2. Phase space reconstruction theory

3.2.1. Phase space reconstruction

Phase space reconstruction is generally the first step of chaotic time series analysis from a time series data. The dynamic characteristic of the system can be explored through phase space reconstruction of the original time series so that the mechanism of the original system can be revealed from the original time series[20]. It has been proved by the so-called Takens' embedding theorem[21]. According to the theorem, the reconstructed phase space can maintain the invariance of geometry for the original dynamical system[22], such as the characteristic value of the fixed point, the fractal dimension of the attractor, the Lyapunov exponent in the phase space orbit, and so on.

Definition 1: Let (N, ρ) and (N_1, ρ_1) as two metric spaces. If the mapping $\varphi : N \to N_1$ satisfies ① φ is a surjection; ② $\rho(x, y) = \rho_1(\varphi x, \varphi y)$, then (N, ρ) and (N_1, ρ_1) are called as the isometric isomorphism.

Definition 2: If (N_1, ρ_1) is isometric isomorphism with a subspace (N_0, ρ_2) of another metric space (N_2, ρ_2), then (N_1, ρ_1) can be embedded into (N_2, ρ_2).

Theorem 1: Let M be a compact manifold of dimension m. For pairs (φ, x), $\varphi : M \to M$ a smooth diffeomorphism and $x : M \to R$ a smooth function, it is a generic property that the map $\phi_{(\varphi, x)} : M \to R^{2m+1}$ is an embedding, where $\phi_{(\varphi, x)}(y) = \{x(y), x(\varphi(y)), \cdots, x(\varphi^{2m}(y))\}$.

In terms of the above definitions and theorem, $\phi_{(\varphi, x)}(y) = \{x(y), x(\varphi(y)), \cdots, x(\varphi^{2m}(y))\}$ is a subspace of R^{2m+1}. $\phi_{(\varphi, x)}$ and the subspace are isometric isomorphic. Then the manifold M of dimension m can be embedded into R^{2m+1}. In other words, $\phi_{(\varphi, x)}$ is an embedding of

$M \to R^{2m+1}$. For a practical time series $\{x_t\}$, the state of the original system is equivalent to the m-dimensional manifold M. In fact, $\{x_t\}$ is a signal observed in the m-dimensional manifold M. If let $\varphi : y_t \to y_{t-\tau_d}$, φ is a smooth diffeomorphism. y_t denotes the state of the system M at time t. τ_d is the delay time. The signal observed in M at time t consist of $\{x_t, x_{t-\tau_d}, \cdots, x_{t-2m\tau_d}\}$, where $x_t = x(y_t)$, $x_{t-\tau} = x(y_{t-\tau_d}) = x(\varphi(y))$, $\cdots$, $x_{t-2m\tau_d} = x(\varphi^{2m}(y))$. $\phi_{(\varphi, x)} = (x_t, x_{t-\tau_d}, \cdots, x_{t-2m\tau_d})$ is an embedding of $M \to R^{2m+1}$. The manifold M is diffeomorphic with $\{x_t, x_{t-\tau_d}, \cdots, x_{t-2m\tau_d}\}$. If the embedding dimension is greater than 2 times the dimension m of the attractor of the original system, the phase space with the base of the practical signal delay time coordinates is equivalent to the state space of the original system. That is, Takens' embedding theorem states that if the time series is indeed composed of scalar measurements of the state from a dynamical system, then under certain genericity assumptions, a one-to-one image of the original set $\{x\}$ is given by the time-delay embedding, provided d is large enough. At present, the delay coordinate method has been widely used to give the phase space reconstruction from the original signal.

For a time series $x(t)$ observed by the measure function h, i.e.

$$x(t) = h(Y) \tag{24}$$

the vector $\overline{X}_t$ can be constructed as follows,

$$\overline{X}_t = (x(t), x(t - \tau_d), x(t - 2\tau_d), \cdots, x(t - (d-1)\tau_d))^T \tag{25}$$

where τ_d is an integer multiple of the sampling interval τ, called as the lag time or delay time. d is and embedding dimension, $d \geq 2m+1$. m is an attractor dimension of the original system.

3.2.2. Problems in phase space reconstruction

Takens' embedding theorem offers in the absence of noise, the possibility of reconstructing n-dimensional dynamics from one-dimensional infinite data of one observable-measurable system. This means that in the case of any delay time, a time series can always be embedded into the state space of the system, and when the embedding dimension is sufficiently large, reconstructed space and embedded space is almost one-to-one correspondence. Therefore, one can reconstruct a phase space from an experimental time series so as to estimate dynamical invariants of the time series, such as dimensions, Lyapunov exponents, entropies[21, 23, 24] and so on. However, the embedding theorem does not directly answer how to choose embedding dimension d and delay time t. In practical application, the experimental data is always limited and noisy so that the estimation of the above parameters presents some difficulties[25, 26]. Accuracy of the phase space reconstruction is critically important to the estimation of invariant measures characterizing system behavior. The choice of delay time τ_d and embedding dimension d always has a great impact on the phase space reconstruction.

Some researchers have studied the choice of delay time τ_d [26-30]. If the delay time τ_d is too small, the reconstructed attractor will be crowded around the main diagonal, which is called as redundance. If τ_d is too large, the dynamic shape of the attractor will be broken, which is called as irrelevance, and the phase space reconstruction is no longer representative of the true dynamics in the real system[28]. In normal circumstances, in order to make the elements of $\overline{Y}_t$ independent, τ_d is the same for all the embedding dimension d[27-29]. The autocorrelation function method and mutual information technique[30] have been most commonly used to give the delay time τ_d although the issue of the delay time choice has still been completely resolved.

For the embedding dimension d, there are three methods that are usually used to choose the appropriate embedding dimension, including the correlation dimension, singular value decomposition(SVD), the false neighbors[21, 31, 32]. The correlation dimension method is to estimate appropriate dimension d in terms of the correlation theorem[8, 21, 33]. By increasing the embedding dimension, one notes an appropriate dimension d when the value of the correlation dimension stops changing. Broomhead and King[31] used the singular value decomposition (SVD) technique to determine an appropriate embedding dimension d directly from the raw time series. The false neighbor method is based on the fact that choosing a too low embedding dimension results in points, which are far apart in the original phase space, being moved closer together in the reconstruction space[32]. Besides, there are also some other methods and modified extensions developed based on the above methods. However, there are still problems on how to determine the appropriate embedding dimension from a scalar time series[34-38].

3.3. Correlation dimension

If a system is chaotic, the strange attractor in a region of the phase space constitutes an infinite hierarchy of self-similar structure, i.e. a fractal structure. One can use quantitative measures to define the fractal nature. The correlation dimension is a useful measurement. Grassberger and Proccacia give a kind of computation method, called GP algorithm[33, 39, 40].

3.3.1. GP algorithm of correlation dimension

Let $X_1, X_2, ..., X_n$ be a point of the attractor in phase space. $C_l(X_j)$ is denoted as a hypersurface sphere with the radius l at the reference point X_j. $\mu[C_l(X_i)]$ is the probability that X_i ($i=1, ..., n$) falls into $C_l(X_j)$, as follows.

$$\mu[C_l(X_j)] = \frac{1}{n}\sum_{i=1}^{n}\theta(l - \|X_i - X_j\|) \tag{26}$$

where $\|\bullet\|$ is Euclidean norm. $\theta(r)$ is Heaviside function whose value is 1 if $r \geq 0$, otherwise, zero.

Then a correlation integral function is defined as

$$C(l) = \frac{1}{n^2} \sum_{i=1}^{n} \sum_{j=1}^{n} \theta(l - \|X_i - X_j\|) \tag{27}$$

with $l \to 0$, there are a scaling relation $C(l) \propto l^{D_2}$ between the correlation integral $C(l)$ and l. A correlation dimension D_2 is defined.

$$D_2 = \lim_{l \to 0} \frac{\ln C(l)}{\ln(l)} \tag{28}$$

In practical computation, D_2 is the slope of log C vs log l curve over a selected straight line range.

3.3.2. Correlation dimension theorem[41]

Theorem 2: Let a map $G : R^n \to R^n$. A is an attractor of map G that has only a finite number of periodic points of period P. Under a natural probability measure μ, the correlation dimension of A is $D_2(\mu)$. For a measure function h of A, $h : R^n \to R$, define a delay coordinate map $F_h : R^n \to R^d$ as

$$F_h(X) = [h(X), h(G^{-1}(X)), \cdots, h(G^{-(d-1)}(X))] \tag{29}$$

where $d \geq P$. $F_h(\mu)$ is a natural probability measure in R^d of $F_h(A)$. If $d \geq D_2(\mu)$, then for almost every h, $D_2(F_h(\mu)) = D_2(\mu)$.

The theorem says that with the embedding dimension increasing, the slope of corresponding correlation integral curve will converge to the correlation dimension D_2 of the original system attractor. Therefore, the optimal embedding dimension can be estimated by using the correlation dimension D_2. That is, if the embedding dimension $d \geq D_2$, the slope of the correlation integral curve is equal to the correlation dimension. This also indicates that the dimension estimation actually does not have to meet the requirements of the embedding theorem on the embedding dimension $d \geq 2D_2 + 1$. When the embedding dimension $d \geq D_2$, the reconstructed attractor can contain the fractal structural feature of the original system attractor to reflect the chaotic characteristics of the original system. Correlation dimension has been widely used in the analysis of chaotic time series.

3.3.3. Chaotic test based on correlation dimension

Chaos has a fractal structure so that the corresponding correlation dimension D_2 is a fractional value. The estimation of correlation dimension D_2 from a time series can be used to determine whether the time series is chaotic. If D_2 is fractional, the original time series can have chaotic features, otherwise, it cannot be chaotic. According to the correlation dimension theorem, when the embedding dimension d of the reconstructed phase space is increased to a certain value, the correlation dimension D_2 will be saturated. Then, the optimal embedding dimension d will be given from a time series. The corresponding correlation dimension D_2 is called as the correlation dimension of this time series.

Lorenz chaotic time series is given by the state variable x of Lorenz system as follows.

$$\begin{cases} \dfrac{dx}{dt} = \sigma(y - x) \\ \dfrac{dy}{dt} = rx - y - xz \\ \dfrac{dz}{dt} = -bz + xy \end{cases} \tag{30}$$

where $\sigma=10$, $b=8/3$, $r=28$, initial conditions: $x(0)=5$, $y(0)=5$, $z(0)=15$. The sampling interval $\tau=0.1$. The sampling points $N=1000$. For delay time $\tau_d=\tau$, the corresponding correlation dimension values are given in Table 1 when the embedding dimension d is increased from 2 to 12. From this table, we can see that the correlation dimension of the time series is about 2.07. The result shows that the reconstructed attractor has a fractal structure to reflect the chaotic feature of the system. The time series can reconstruct the state space of the original system when the embedding dimension $d=6$.

Logistic chaotic time series $\{x_n\}_{n=1}^{N}$ is given by Logistic system in Eq.16 with $\alpha=3.9$ and $e=0$. The length N is 1000 points. Here, $\tau_d=1$ (i.e. discrete time series interval). With increasing the embedding dimension d, the corresponding correlation dimension is 0.97 (see Table 2). The optimal embedding dimension is 2.

For finite sampling number (e.g. $N=1000$), the reconstructed attractor will be broken when the embedding dimension d is increased continuously to a higher value. The estimation of correlation dimension will fail during computation. Therefore, embedding dimension d should not be unlimitedly increased.

d	2	3	4	5	6	7	8	9	10	11	12
D_2	1.8009	1.9284	1.9718	2.0389	2.0737	2.0966	2.086	2.0788	2.0705	2.0760	2.0753

Table 1. The analysis of correlation dimensions of Lorenz chaos time series

d	1	2	3	4	5	6	7	8	9	10	11
D_2	0.9598	0.9718	0.9689	0.9713	0.9718	0.9591	0.9774	0.9621	0.9827	0.9826	0.9839

Table 2. The analysis of correlation dimensions of Logistic chaos time series

3.3.4. The analysis of surface EMG signal based on correlation dimension

From the above analysis, we can see that the surface EMG signal has deterministic nonlinear component. Here, the correlation dimension is further used to study whether its nonlinear component are chaotic. Figure 10a shows a raw data for forearm pronation. Figure 10b gives the correlation integral curve of the data under the embedding dimension from 2 to 12. In the recontructed phase space, the delay time τ_d is chosen as the sampling interval. With the increase of embedding dimension, the straight line segments of the computed correlation integral curves will tend to be parallel and keep unchange in the range.

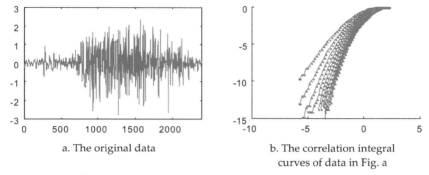

a. The original data

b. The correlation integral
curves of data in Fig. a

Figure 10. The correlation dimension analysis of surface EMG signal

The corresponding slope value is the correlation dimension of the surface EMG signal, about 3.8050 ± 0.0560 (see Table 3). The result indicates that the surface EMG signal during movement has fractal feature to reveal the implied chaotic motion behavior. Table 3 shows that the reconstructed attractor contains the nature of the raw system when the embedding dimension is over 6.

d	2	3	4	5	6	7	8	9	10	11	12
D_2	1.9315	2.7037	3.2808	3.4837	3.8047	3.7597	3.8511	3.8864	3.8129	3.7160	3.8039

Table 3. The analysis of correlation dimension of surface EMG signal during movement

3.3.5. Study of surrogate data test method based on correlation dimension

The correlation dimension is a quantitative index that describes the fractal structure of chaotic attractor. It measures the freedom degree and complexity of the system. For the raw data and all data of $F \in F_\phi$, in the case of the same embedding dimension, the corresponding test results will be obviously significant[42]. Here, the correlation dimension is used as a test statistic to analyze the surface EMG signal. According to the null hypothesis 3, 39 sets of surrogate data are produced in confidence level 95%. In order to quickly obtain the correlation dimension in a variety of circumstances, the linear parts of all correlation integral curves are taken as the same. Though these values are not accurate, this test algorithm is great effective to test the chaotic fractal feature of the experimental data.

When the sampling interval τ=1, Figure 11a and b show the results of the surrogate data test analysis for Lorenz chaotic time series based on correlation dimension. There are significant differences between the original data and its surrogate data in m = 5 (see Fig. 11a). This result explains that the null hypothesis can be rejected in confidence level 95%. The

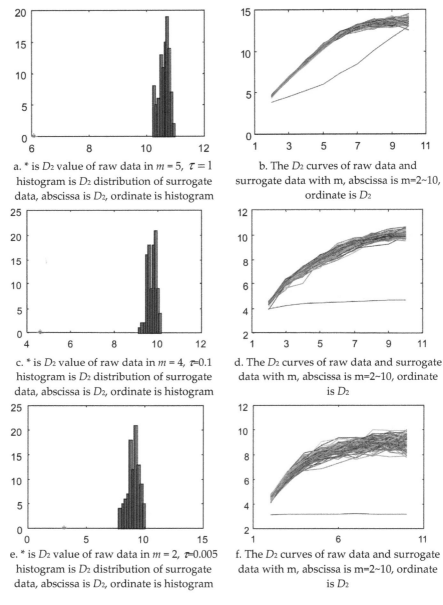

a. * is D_2 value of raw data in $m = 5$, $\tau = 1$ histogram is D_2 distribution of surrogate data, abscissa is D_2, ordinate is histogram

b. The D_2 curves of raw data and surrogate data with m, abscissa is m=2~10, ordinate is D_2

c. * is D_2 value of raw data in $m = 4$, $\tau=0.1$ histogram is D_2 distribution of surrogate data, abscissa is D_2, ordinate is histogram

d. The D_2 curves of raw data and surrogate data with m, abscissa is m=2~10, ordinate is D_2

e. * is D_2 value of raw data in $m = 2$, $\tau=0.005$ histogram is D_2 distribution of surrogate data, abscissa is D_2, ordinate is histogram

f. The D_2 curves of raw data and surrogate data with m, abscissa is m=2~10, ordinate is D_2

Figure 11. The surrogate data test analysis based on correlation dimension for Lorenz chaos time series by sampling intervals

differences disappear between the raw data and its surrogate data in $m = 10$ (see Fig. 11b). This illustrates that the reconstructed attractor appears broken. The reconstructed phase space is similar to that of the surrogate data with linear stochastic noise characteristics.

Figure 11c and d show the results with τ=0.1. The differences between the raw data and its surrogate data can be seen in Fig. 11c ($m = 4$). When m>2, these differences become larger as m increases. Figure 11e and f show the results with τ=0.005. Figure 11e shows the surrogate data test histogram in $m = 2$. The correlation dimension curves of the raw data and its surrogate data are given in $m = 2 \sim 10$ (see Fig. 11f). Even in the case of oversampling, the correlation dimension as test statistic can also make the surrogate data method very effective.

3.3.6. The surface EMG signal analysis based on the surrogate data and correlation dimension

Figure 12 shows the surrogate data analysis for the surface EMG signal in Fig. 12a based on correlation dimension. When $m = 6$, the correlation dimension value of the raw data is different from those of its surrogate data generated by the null hypothesis 3. The correlation dimension curves of the raw data and its surrogate data are given when $m = 2 \sim 8$ in Fig. 12b. We can see the differences between the original data and its surrogate data. The null hypothesis 3 can be rejected in confidence level 95%. The result indicates that the surface EMG signal has deterministic nonlinear components, even chaotic.

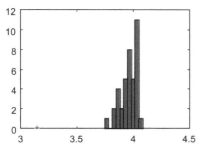
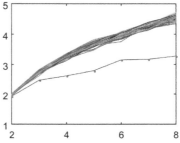

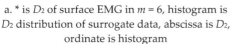

a. * is D_2 of surface EMG in $m = 6$, histogram is D_2 distribution of surrogate data, abscissa is D_2, ordinate is histogram

b. The curves of surface EMG and surrogate data with m, abscissa is m=2~8, ordinate is D_2

Figure 12. The surrogate data test analysis based on correlation dimension for surface EMG signal.

3.4. Largest Lyapunov exponent

The Lyapunov exponent method is to directly identify whether a system is chaotic. If the system is chaotic, the Lyapunov exponent is positive. Otherwise, the Lyapunov exponent is negative. For this, the Lyapunov exponent can be used to test the chaotic feature of a signal under study. The first algorithms developed computed the whole Lyapunov spectrum by

Wolf et al. [43] and Sano et al. [44]. Meanwhile, the largest Lyapunov exponent is sufficient for assessing the presence of chaos. At present, there are many algorithms to estimate the largest Lyapunov exponent from a time series, such as an algorithm given by Rosenstein et al.[45]. This algorithm is aimed specifically at estimating the largest Lyapunov exponent from short data.

3.4.1. Algorithm of largest Lyapunov exponent estimation[45]

For a short time series, Rosenstein et al. present a robust estimation algorithm of the largest Lyapunov exponent. First, the attractor is reconstructed, refer to Eq. 25. Next, the algorithm locates the closest neighbor of each point X_i on the trajectory, with respect to the Euclidian distance. Then, one defines the distance between two neighboring points at instant $n=0$ by:

$$d_i(0) = \min_{X_j} \|X_j - X_i\| \tag{31}$$

where $\| \bullet \|$ is the Euclidian norm. Here, the temporal separation of the nearest neighbors should be greater than the mean period of the time series.

$$|i - j| > mean\ period \tag{32}$$

According to time, the average distance between two neighboring vectors can be simply

$$d_i(n) = \|X_{j+n} - X_{i+n}\| \tag{33}$$

Assume that the system is controlled by the largest Lyapunov exponent only. Then, the distance between two neighbor points obey the following relationship:

$$d(t) = Ce^{\lambda t} \tag{34}$$

For $t = n\Delta t$, there is:

$$d_i(n) \approx C_i e^{\lambda n \Delta t} \tag{35}$$

$$\lambda = \frac{1}{n \cdot \Delta t} \ln \frac{d_i(n)}{C_i} \tag{36}$$

$$n \cdot \lambda = \frac{1}{\Delta t}(\ln d_i(n) - \ln C_i) \tag{37}$$

$$n\langle \lambda \rangle = \frac{1}{\Delta t}\langle \ln d_i(n)\rangle - \frac{1}{\Delta t}\langle \ln C_i \rangle$$
$$= \frac{1}{\Delta t}\langle \ln d_i(n)\rangle - b \tag{38}$$

where $b = \frac{1}{\Delta t}\langle \ln C_i \rangle$.

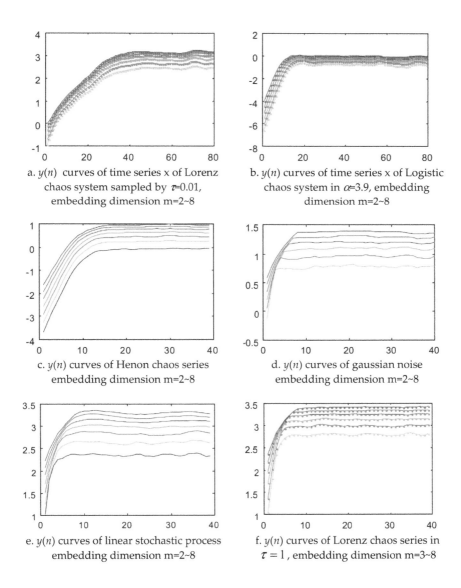

a. $y(n)$ curves of time series x of Lorenz chaos system sampled by τ=0.01, embedding dimension m=2~8

b. $y(n)$ curves of time series x of Logistic chaos system in α=3.9, embedding dimension m=2~8

c. $y(n)$ curves of Henon chaos series embedding dimension m=2~8

d. $y(n)$ curves of gaussian noise embedding dimension m=2~8

e. $y(n)$ curves of linear stochastic process embedding dimension m=2~8

f. $y(n)$ curves of Lorenz chaos series in $\tau = 1$, embedding dimension m=3~8

Figure 13. $y(n)$ curves of signals, abscissa is n, ordinate is $y(n)$

Then, the Lyapunov exponent can be given by using a least-squares fit to the "average" line:

$$y(n) = \frac{1}{\Delta t}\langle \ln d_i(n) \rangle \tag{39}$$

where $y(n) = n\langle \lambda \rangle + b$. The largest Lyapunov exponent λ is the slope of $y(n)$ in the above equation.

This method is deduced directly from the largest Lyapunov exponent definition. The accurate evaluation of λ depends on the full use of the data. In practice, the curve $y(n)$ will tend to saturation. The largest Lyapunov exponent λ is given by computing the slope of the linear part in the curve $y(n)$.

3.4.2. Chaos test based on largest Lyapunov exponent

In general, if the signal is chaotic, the slope of the curve $y(n)$ will be independent of the embedding dimension. Otherwise, if the signal is not chaotic, the slope of the curve $y(n)$ will depend on the embedding dimension. When the embedding dimension m is chosen from 2 to 8, the Lyapunov exponent of the curve $y(n)$ of the signal is shown in Figure 13. For a chaotic signal, a good illustration is given (see Figure 13a, b and c). The $y(n)$ curves are different from those of a non-chaotic signal (compare with Figure 13d and e). However, even for chaotic signals, the $y(n)$ curves are not always parallel. For example, in the case of undersampling ($\tau = 1$), the $y(n)$ curves of Lorenz chaotic time series are similar to those of linear stochastic process(compare with Figure 13e and f). In the literature[23], the $y(n)$ curves of the Ikeda chaotic time series are also not parallel.

3.4.3. The analysis of surface EMG signal based on the largest Lyapunov exponent

Figure 14 gives the curves of Lyapunove exponent $y(n)$ for the surface EMG signal. The $y(n)$ curves are not very parallel for the surface EMG signal. It is difficult to distinguish the curves of $y(n)$ for the surface EMG signal from those of Figure 13d, f and g. The surface EMG signal can not be determined as chaotic, or as stochastic. But it can be a high-dimensional system.

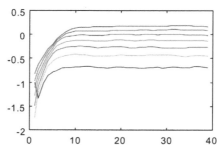

Figure 14. $y(n)$ curves of surface EMG signal, embedding dimension m=2~8, abscissa is n, ordinate is $y(n)$

3.5. Principal component analysis

Broomhead and King[31] proposed the idea of singular system analysis that determines an appropriate embedding dimension d directly from the raw time series. It provides its convenience for the further analysis of the given system. Numerical experience, however, led several authors to express some doubts about reliability of singular system analysis in the attractor reconstruction[46-48]. Palus and Dvorak[37] explain why singular-value decomposition(SVD), the heart of the singular system analysis and by nature a linear method, may become misleading technique when it is used in nonlinear dynamics studies that reconstruction parameters are time-delay, embedding dimension (or embedding windows). For this, we propose a novel nonlinear analysis method based symplectic geometry, called symplectic principal component analysis(SPCA)[49].

3.5.1. Principle and algorithm of principal component analysis

Let a time series $x_1, x_2,..., x_n$ be the measured signal by sampling interval t_s, n is the number of samples. According to Takens' embedding theorem, a trajectory matrix X can be given by time delay coordinates method, refer to Eq. 25(τ_d=1):

$$X = \begin{bmatrix} X_1^T \\ X_2^T \\ \vdots \\ X_m^T \end{bmatrix} = \begin{bmatrix} x_1 & x_2 & \cdots & x_d \\ x_2 & x_3 & \cdots & x_{d+1} \\ \vdots & \vdots & \cdots & \vdots \\ x_m & x_{m+1} & \cdots & x_n \end{bmatrix} \tag{40}$$

where d is embedding dimension. $m=n-d+1$ is the number of points in d-dimension reconstruction attractor, $X_i^T, i = 1, \cdots\cdots, m$, denotes a point in the attractor. For the matrix X, there are a $m\times d$ orthogonal matrix V and a $d\times d$ orthogonal matrix. The matrix X can be decomposed as follows.

$$X = VSU^T \tag{41}$$

where S is $d\times d$ diagonal matrix, whose elements are defined

$$S_{ij} = \delta_{ij}\sqrt{\sigma_i m}, \qquad i, j = 1, 2, \cdots, d \tag{42}$$

Since the matrix V is orthogonal, then

$$(V^T \cdot V)_{ij} = \delta_{ij} \tag{43}$$

Meanwhile, for the matrix U, there are

$$(U^T \cdot U)_{ij} = (U \cdot U^T)_{ij} = \delta_{ij} \tag{44}$$

In order to facilitate the calculation, Broomhead et al. applies the covariance matrix C of the matrix X to replace the matrix X. The details are as follows:

$$C = \frac{1}{m} \cdot X^T \cdot X \tag{45}$$

$$C_{ij} = \frac{1}{m} \sum_{k=1}^{m} x_{i+k-1} x_{j+k-1} , \qquad i, j = 1, 2, \cdots, d \tag{46}$$

Its values reflect the degree of correlation between the time delay coordinate variable i and j.

$$C = \frac{1}{m} \cdot X^T \cdot X = \frac{1}{m} \cdot U \cdot S \cdot S \cdot U^T = \frac{1}{m} \cdot U \cdot S^2 \cdot U^T \tag{47}$$

$$U^T \cdot C \cdot U = \frac{1}{m} \cdot (XU)^T \cdot XU = \frac{1}{m} \cdot S^2 \tag{48}$$

Let $Y=XU$, then:

$$U^T \cdot C \cdot U = \frac{1}{m} \cdot Y^T \cdot Y = \frac{1}{m} \cdot S^2 \tag{49}$$

where $U^T C U$ is the covariance matrix of the matrix Y. Its elements are zero, except that the diagonal elements are equal to σ_i. This means that the variables i and j of the matrix Y are independent. The coordinate system is orthogonal, which is constituted from the variables of the matrix Y after the above transformed. The σ_i is called the principal component or singular value in accordance with the order of the largest to the smallest. The orthogonal vector U_i corresponding to the principal component σ_i is called the principal axis. The principal component describes the distribution of the signal energy. That is, the value of the principal component reflects the projection of the signal energy in the corresponding principal axis. In the different principal axes, a distribution value is given as $\sigma_i / \sum_{i=1}^{d} \sigma_i$, where $\sum_{i=1}^{d} \sigma_i$ is the total energy of the signal. If $\sigma_{i+1} \approx \cdots \approx \sigma_d$, the distribution values are called a noise floor. The distribution can be used to estimate the dimension of the dynamical system that generates a time series or to filter out the noise. Let $\overline{U}_i$ be the principal axes corresponding to the principal components over the noise floor. Zero vector describes the principal axes corresponding to the noise floor. Thus, for σ_i > noise floor, a new coordinate transform matrix is made up of:

$$\overline{U} = [\overline{U}_1, \overline{U}_2, \cdots, \overline{U}_i, 0, \cdots, 0] \tag{50}$$

In order to filter out noise, the trajectory matrix X is first projected into the coordinate system U.

$$Y = XU \tag{51}$$

The variables in the matrix Y are independent. Then, the original coordinate system is updated by using the matrix Y:

$$\overline{X} = Y\overline{U}^T = (XU) \cdot \overline{U}^T \tag{52}$$

That is, $\overline{X}$ is a new time delay coordinate system.

3.5.2. Influence of noise on the principal component spectrum of chaotic time series

Figure 15a shows the principal component spectrum of Logistic attractor from a Logistic chaotic time series without noise. The principal component spectrum has not a significant noise level. When the interior noise is Gaussian noise with zero mean and 0.001^2 variance, the principal component spectrum is given for Logistic attractor. Figure 15c and d give the principal component spectrum of Logistic attractor with the measurement noise $\sigma^2=0.001^2$ and $\sigma^2=0.8^2$, respectively. It can be seen that the Logistic attractor with the internal noise has the same principal component spectrum as the attractor without noise. The curves of the principal component spectrum are also slanting. The total energy is significantly distributed into each principal axes. The principal components are declining with the index i so that there is no noise floor. It is difficult to choose an appropriate embedding dimension d. For the larger measurement noise, the corresponding principal component spectrum of Logistic attractor slant into a floor area with increasing the embedding dimension. In the floor area, the principal components keep unchanged and do not decline with the index i, called noise floor. Broomhead and King[31] have suggested that this noise floor can be used to determine the embedding dimension and filter out noise from the data. The signal energy will be focused on the truncated principal components and the corresponding principal axes

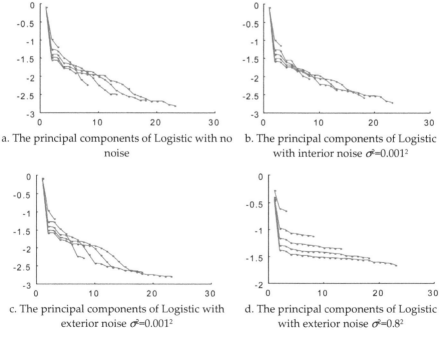

a. The principal components of Logistic with no noise

b. The principal components of Logistic with interior noise $\sigma^2=0.001^2$

c. The principal components of Logistic with exterior noise $\sigma^2=0.001^2$

d. The principal components of Logistic with exterior noise $\sigma^2=0.8^2$

Figure 15. The principal component analysis of Logistic chaos series with different noises based on SVD, d=3 : 2 : 23, abscissa is d, ordinate is $\log(\sigma_i / tr(\sigma_i))$

when the principal components above noise floor are only held. The number of the principal components above the noise floor is the optimal embedding dimension.

Besides, the new coordinate system corresponding to the principal axes can eliminate the noise floor to reduce the noise from the data. However, the truncated position of the principal components depends on the signal-noise-ratio, especially for the measurement noise. The principal components of the chaotic time series based on SVD spectrum more easily subject to the measurement noise so that the embedding dimension estimation is directly affected. For the smaller noise, there is the more number of principal components above the noise floor. For the larger noise, the number of the corresponding principal components will be reduced. Here, the above calculation accuracy is 2.2204e-016, which does not consider the numerical calculation error.

3.5.3. Influence of sampling interval on the principal component spectrum of chaotic time series[49]

The Lorenz chaotic system is considered to give the state variable x in order to study the influence of sampling interval on the principal component spectrum. The principal component spectrum slant and have no floor for the chaotic time series x with $\tau=0.005$ (see Fig. 16a). When $\tau=0.1$ (see Fig. 16b), the principal component spectrum are basically similar

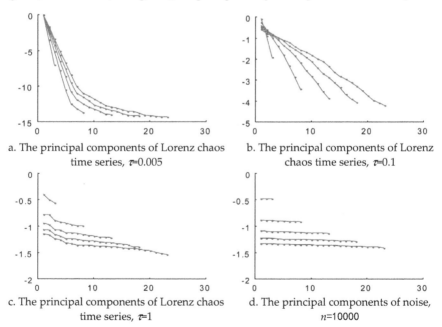

a. The principal components of Lorenz chaos time series, $\tau=0.005$

b. The principal components of Lorenz chaos time series, $\tau=0.1$

c. The principal components of Lorenz chaos time series, $\tau=1$

d. The principal components of noise, $n=10000$

Figure 16. The principal component analysis of gaussian noise and Lorenz chaos time series by different sampling intervals based on SVD, $d=3:2:23$, abscissa is d, ordinate is $\log(\sigma_i / tr(\sigma_i))$

to those in the Figure 16a. When τ=1, each line is separated from each other and tends to horizontal line in the case of different embedding dimensions(see Fig. 16c). It shows that the distribution of the total energy has little difference in each principal axis, like the Gaussian noise (see Fig. 16d). For the Gaussian noise, its principal component spectrum curves are horizontal lines, where N=10000. It shows that every principal component is equal to each other. The energy distributes into every principal axis averagely. Therefore, it can be seen that sampling interval affects the determination of embedding dimension. When the sampling interval is not undersampling, the determination of embedding dimension depends the amount of signal-noise-ratio. In the case of undersampling, the chaotic time series is similar to noise so that the embedding dimension seems to be estimated as 1.

3.6. Symplectic principal component analysis

The symplectic geometry is a kind of phase space geometry. Its nature is nonlinear. It can describe the system structure, especially nonlinear structure, very well. It has been used to study various nonlinear dynamical systems[50-52] since Feng Kang[53] has proposed a symplectic algorithm for solving symplectic differential. However, from the view of data analysis, few literatures have employed symplectic geometry theory to explore the dynamics of the system. Our previous works have proposed the estimation of the embedding dimension based on symplectic geometry from a time series[49, 54-56]. Subsequently, Niu et al. have used our method to evaluate sprinter's surface EMG signals[57]. Xie et al[58] have proposed a kind of symplectic geometry spectra based on our work. Subsequently, we show that SPCA can well represent chaotic time series and reduce noise in chaotic data[59, 60].

In SPCA, a fundamental step is to build the multidimensional structure (attractor) in symplectic geometry space. Here, in terms of Taken's embedding theorem, we first construct an attractor in phase space, i.e. the trajectory matrix X from a time series. That is, for a measured data (the observable of the system under study) x_1, x_2, ..., x_n recorded with sampling interval t_s, the corresponding d-dimension reconstruction attractor, $X_{m \times d}$ can be given (refer to Eq.40).Then we describe the symplectic principal component analysis (SPCA) based on symplectic geometry theory and give its corresponding algorithm.

3.7. Symplectic principal component method

SPCA is a kind of PCA approaches based on symplectic geometry. Its idea is to map the investigated complex system in symplectic space and elucidate the dominant features underlying the measured data. The first few larger components capture the main relationship between the variables in symplectic space. The remaining components are composed of the less important components or noise in the measured data. In symplectic space, the used geometry is called symplectic geometry. Different from Eulid geometry, symplectic geometry is the even dimensional geometry with a special symplectic structure. It is dependent on a bilinear antisymmetric nonsingular cross product——symplectic cross product:

$$[x, y] = \langle x, Jy \rangle \tag{53}$$

$$\text{where,} \quad J = J_{2n} = \begin{bmatrix} 0 & +I_n \\ -I_n & 0 \end{bmatrix} \tag{54}$$

When $n = 1$, $x = [x_1, x_2]$, $y = [y_1, y_2]$,

$$J = \begin{bmatrix} 0 & 1 \\ -1 & 0 \end{bmatrix} \tag{55}$$

$$[x, y] = [x_1 \; x_2] J \begin{bmatrix} y_1 \\ y_2 \end{bmatrix}$$

$$= \begin{vmatrix} x_1 & y_1 \\ x_2 & y_2 \end{vmatrix} \tag{56}$$

The measurement of symplectic space is area scale. In symplectic space, the length of arbitrary vectors always equals zero and without signification, and there is the concept of orthogonal cross-course. In symplectic geometry, the symplectic transform is the nonlinear transform in essence, which is also called canonical transform, since it has measure preserving characteristics and can keep the natural properties of the original data unchanged. It is fit for nonlinear dynamics systems.

The symplectic principal components are given by symplectic similar transform. It is similar to SVD-based PCA. The corresponding eigenvalues can be obtained by symplectic QR method. Here, we first construct the autocorrelation matrix $A_{d \times d}$ of the trajectory matrix $X_{m \times d}$. Then the matrix A can be transformed as a Hamilton matrix M in symplectic space.

Definition 1 Let S is a matrix, if $JSJ^{-1} = S^{-*}$, then S is a symplectic matrix.

Definition 2 Let H is a matrix, if $JHJ^{-1} = -H^*$, then H is a Hamilton matrix.

Theorem 1 Any $d \times d$ matrix can be made into a Hamilton matrix. Let a matrix as A, so $\begin{pmatrix} A & 0 \\ 0 & -A^T \end{pmatrix}$ is a Hamilton matrix. (Proof refers to appendix A)

Theorem 2 Hamilton matrix M keeps unchanged at symplectic similar transform. (Proof refers to appendix A)

Theorem 3 Let $M \in C^{2d \times 2d}$ as Hamilton matrix, so e^M is symplectic matrix.

Theorem 4 Let $S \in C^{2d \times 2d}$ as symplectic matrix, there is $S = QR$, where Q is symplectic unitary matrix, R is upper triangle matrix.

Theorem 5 The product of sympletcic matrixes is also a symplectic matrix. (Proof refers to appendix A)

Theorem 6 Suppose Household matrix H is :

$$H = H(k,\omega) = \begin{pmatrix} P & 0 \\ 0 & P \end{pmatrix} \qquad (57)$$

where $P = I_n - \dfrac{2\varpi\varpi^*}{\varpi^*\varpi}$, $\varpi = (0,\cdots,0;\omega_k,\cdots,\omega_d)^T \neq 0$

so, H is symplectic unitary matrix. ϖ^* is ϖ conjugate transposition. (Proof refers to appendix A)

For Hamilton matrix M , its eigenvalues can be given by symplectic similar transform and the primary $2d$ dimension space can be transformed into d dimension space to resolve[17-19], as follows:

i.   Let $N = M^2$

$$M^2 = \begin{bmatrix} A^T & G \\ F & -A \end{bmatrix}^2 \qquad (58)$$

ii. Construct a symplectic matrix Q,

$$Q^T NQ = \begin{bmatrix} B & R \\ 0 & B^T \end{bmatrix} \qquad (59)$$

where B is up Hessenberg matrix ($b_{ij}=0$, $i>j+1$). The matrix Q may be a symplectic Household matrix H. If the matrix M is a real symmetry matrix, M can be considered as N. Then one can get an upper Hessenberg matrix (referred to equ. 13), namely,

$$\begin{aligned}
HMH' &= \begin{pmatrix} P & 0 \\ 0 & P \end{pmatrix}\begin{pmatrix} A & 0 \\ 0 & -A' \end{pmatrix}\begin{pmatrix} P & 0 \\ 0 & P \end{pmatrix}' \\
&= \begin{pmatrix} PAP' & 0 \\ 0 & -PA'P' \end{pmatrix} \\
&= \begin{pmatrix} B & 0 \\ 0 & -B' \end{pmatrix}
\end{aligned} \qquad (60)$$

where H is the symplectic Householder matrix.

iii. Calculate eigenvalues $\lambda(B) = \{\mu_1, \mu_2, \cdots, \mu_d\}$ by using symplectic QR decomposition method; if M is a real symmetry matrix, the eigenvalues of A is equal to those of B:

$$\mu = \lambda(B) = \lambda(A) \qquad (61)$$

$$\lambda(A) = \lambda^2(X) \qquad (62)$$

iv. These eigenvalues $\mu = \{\mu_1, \mu_2, \cdots, \mu_d\}$ are sorted by descending order, that is

$$\mu_1 > \mu_2 > \cdots > \mu_k >> \mu_{k+1} \geq \cdots \geq \mu_d \qquad (63)$$

Thus the calculation of $2d$ dimension space is transformed into that of that of d dimension space. The μ is the symplectic principal component spectrums of A with relevant symplectic orthonormal bases. In the so-called noise floor, values of μ_i, $i = k+1, \cdots, d$, reflect the noise level in the data[49, 55]. The corresponding matrix Q denotes symplectic eigenvectors of A.

3.7.1. Proposed algorithm of symplectic principal component method

For a measured data $x_1, x_2, \ldots, x_n$, our proposed algorithm consists of the following steps:

1. Reconstruct the attractor $X_{m \times d}$ from the measured time series, where d is the embedding dimension of the matrix X, and $m = n-d+1$.
2. Remove the mean values X_{mean} of each row of the matrix X.
3. Build the real $d \times d$ symmetry matrix A, that is,

$$A = (X - X_{mean})'(X - X_{mean}) \tag{64}$$

   Here, d should be larger than the dimension of the system in terms of Taken's embedding theorem.

4. Calculate the symplectic principal components of the matrix A by QR decomposition, and choose the Householder matrix H instead of the transform matrix Q. It is easy to prove that H is a symplectic unitary matrix (Proof refers to appendix A) and H can be constructed from real matrix (refer to appendix B).
5. Construct the corresponding principal eigenvalue matrix W according to the number k of the chosen symplectic principal components of the matrix A, where $W \subseteq Q$. That is, when $k=d$, $W=Q$, otherwise $W \subset Q$. In use, k can be chosen according to Eq.63.
6. Get the transformed coefficients $S = \{S_1, S_2, \ldots, S_m\}$, where

$$S_i = W'X_i, \quad i = 1, \cdots, m \tag{65}$$

7. Reestimate the X_s from S,

$$X_{si} = WS_i \tag{66}$$

   Then the reestimation data $x_{s1}, x_{s2}, \cdots, x_{sm}$ can be given.

8. For the noisy time series, the first estimation of data is usually not good. Here, one can go back to the step (6) and let $X_i = X_s$ in Eq.(65) to do step (6) and (7) again. Generally, the second estimated data will be better than the first estimated data.

Besides, it is necessary to note that for the clean time series, the step (8) is unnecessary to handle.

3.7.2. Performance evaluation

SPCA, like PCA, can not only represent the original data by capturing the relationship between the variables, but also reduce the contribution of errors in the original data. Here, the performance analysis of SPCA is studied from the two views, i.e. representation of chaotic signals and noise reduction in chaotic signals.

Representation of chaotic signals

We first show that for the clean chaotic time series, SPCA can perfectly reconstruct the original data in a high-dimensional space. We first embed the original time series to a phase space. Considering the dimension of the Lorenz system(see Eq. 30) is 3, *d* of the matrix *A* is chosen as 8 in our SPCA analysis. To quantify the difference between the original data and the SPCA-filtered data, we employ the root-mean-square error (RMSE) as a measure:

$$RMSE = \sqrt{\frac{1}{N}\sum_{i=1}^{N}[x(i) - \hat{x}(i)]^2} \qquad (67)$$

where $x(i)$ and $\hat{x}(i)$ are the original data and estimated data, respectively.

When $k = d$, the RMSE values are lower than 10^{-14} (see Figure 17). In Figure 17, the original data are generated by Eq. 30. The estimated data is obtained by SPCA with $k=d$. The results show that the SPCA method is better than the PCA. Since the real systems are usually unknown, it is necessary to study the effect of sampling time, data length, and noise to the SPCA approach. From the Figure 17 and 18, we can see that the sampling time and data length have less effect on SPCA method in the case of free-noise.

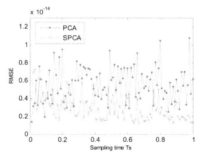

Figure 17. (Color online) RMSE vs. Sampling time curves for the SPCA and PCA.

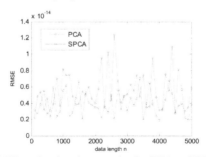

Figure 18. (Color online) RMSE vs. data length curves for the SPCA and PCA.

For analyzing noisy data, we use the percentage of principal components (PCs) to study the occupancy rate of each PC in order to reduce noise. The percentage of PCs is defined by

$$P_i = \frac{\mu_i}{\sum\limits_{i=1}^{d} \mu_i} \times 100\% \qquad (68)$$

where d is the embedding dimension, μ_i is the i-th principal component value. From the Figure 19, we find that the first largest symplectic principal component (SPC) of the SPCA is a little larger than that of the PCA. It is almost possessed of all the proportion of the symplectic principal components. This shows that it is feasible for the SPCA to study the principal component analysis of time series.

Next, we study the reduced space spanned by a few largest symplectic principal components (SPCs) to estimate the chaotic Lorenz time series (see Fig. 20). In Figure 20, the data x is given with a sampling time of 0.01 from chaotic Lorenz system. The estimated data is calculated by the first three largest SPCs. The average error and standard deviation between the original data and the estimated data is -6.55e-16 and 1.03e-2, respectively. The

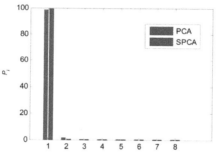

Figure 19. (Color online) The percentage of principal components for the SPCA and PCA.

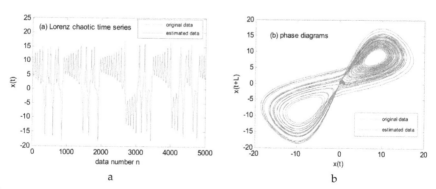

Figure 20. (Colour online) Chaotic signal reconstructed by the proposed SPCA algorithm with k=3, where (a) the time series of the original Lorenz data x without noise and the estimated data; (b) phase diagrams with L =11 for the original Lorenz data x without noise and the estimated data. The sampling time t_s = 0.01.

estimated data is very close to the original data not only in time domain (see Figure 20a) but also in phase space (see Figure 20b). We further explore the effect of sampling time in different number of PCs. When the PCs number k =1 and k =7, respectively, the SPCA and PCA give the change of RMSE values with the sampling time in Figure 21. We can see that the RMSE values of the SPCA are smaller than those of the PCA. The sampling time has less impact on the SPCA than the PCA. In the case of k = 7, the data length has also less effect on the SPCA than the PCA(see Fig. 22).

Comparing with PCA, the results of SPCA are better in the above Figures. We can see that the SPCA method keep the essential dynamical character of the primary time series generated by chaotic continuous systems. These indicate that the SPCA can reflect intrinsic nonlinear characteristics of the original time series. Moreover, the SPCA can elucidate the dominant features underlying the observed data. This will help to retrieve dominant patterns from the noisy data. For this, we study the feasibility of the proposed algorithm to reduce noise by using the noisy chaotic Lorenz data.

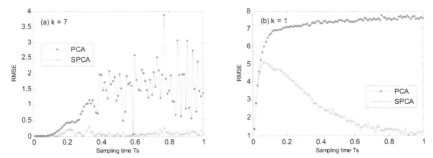

Figure 21. The RMSE values vs. the sampling time for the SPCA and PCA, where (a) the PCs number k =7; (b) k =1.

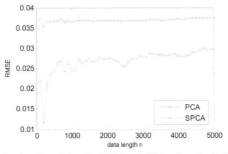

Figure 22. The RMSE vs. the data length for the SPCA and PCA, where k =7. The sampling time is 0.1.

Noise reduction in chaotic signals

For the noisy Lorenz data x, the phase diagrams of the noisy and clean data are given in Figure 23a and 23b. The clean data is the chaotic Lorenz data x with noise-free (see Eq. 30).

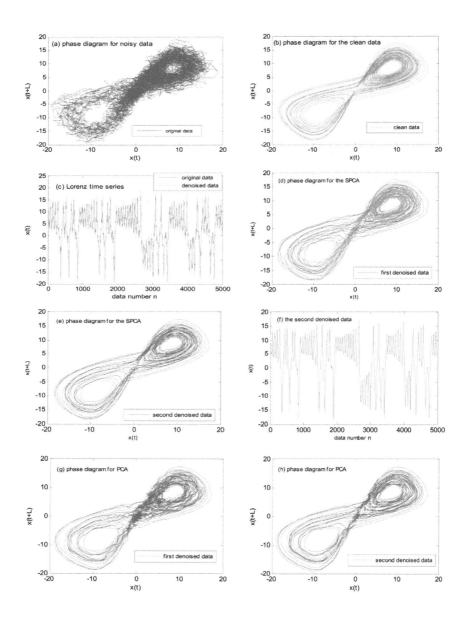

Figure 23. The noise reduction analysis of the proposed SPCA algorithm and PCA for the noisy Lorenz time series, where L=11.

The noisy data is the chaotic Lorenz data x with Gaussian white noise of zero mean and one variance (see Eq. 30). The sampling time is 0.01. The time delay L is 11 in Figure 23. It is obvious that noise is very strong. The first denoised data is obtained in terms of the proposed SPCA algorithm (see Figure 23c- f). Here, we first build an attractor X with the embedding dimension of 8. Then the transform matrix W is constructed when $k=1$. The first denoised data is generated by Eq.(65) and (66). In Figure 23c, the first denoised data is compared with the noisy Lorenz data x from the view of time field. Figure 23d shows the corresponding phase diagram of the first denoised data. Compared with Fig. 23a, the first denoised data can basically give the structure of the original system. In order to obtain better results, this denoised data is reduced noise again by the step (8). We can see that after the second noise reduction, the results are greatly improved in Fig. 23e and 23f, respectively. The curves of the second denoised data are better than those of the first denoised data whether in time domain or in phase space by contrast with Fig. 23c and 23d. Figure 23g shows that the PCA technique gives the first denoised result. We refer to our algorithm to deal with the first denoised data again by the PCA (see Figure 23h). Some of noise has been further reduced but the curve of PCA is not better than that of SPCA in Figure 23e. The reason is that the PCA is a linear method indeed. When nonlinear structures have to be considered, it can be misleading, especially in the case of a large sampling time (see Figure 24). The used program code of the PCA comes from the TISEAN tools (http://www.mpipks–dresden.mpg.de/ ~tisean).

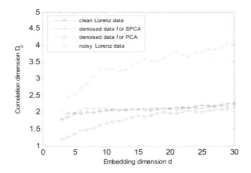

Figure 24. (Color online) D_2 vs. embedding dimension d

Figure 24 shows the variation of correlation dimension D_2 with embedding dimension d in the sampling time of 0.1 for the clean, noisy, and denoised Lorenz data. We can observe that for the clean and SPCA denoised data, the trend of the curves tends to smooth in the vicinity of 2. For the noisy data, the trend of the curve is constantly increasing and has no platform. For the PCA denoised data, the trend of the curve is also increasing and trends to a platform with 2. However, this platform is smaller than that of SPCA. It is less effective than the SPCA algorithm. This indicates that it is difficult for the PCA to describe the nonlinear structure of a system, because the correlation dimension D_2 manifests nonlinear properties of chaotic systems. Here, the correlation dimension D_2 is estimated by the Grassberger-Procaccia's algorithm[33, 40].

3.7.3. Estimation of embedding dimension based on symplectic geometry

In terms of Eq. 63, the values of μ_i, $i=k+1$, ..., d, are far smaller than μ_k. These values form a noise floor. Therefore, the embedding dimension of the reconstruction system can be determined by the noise floor. Here, the noise and nonlinear time series are used to investigate the feasibility of the embedding dimension estimation based on symplectic geometry.

For noise (which is generally regarded as Gauss white noise with mean value 0 and variance 1 in practical systems), symplectic geometry spectrums of this noise give the even distribution of its total energy (see Fig. 25a). From this figure, we can see that the symplectic geometry spectrums of noise can reflect the characteristic of noise very well when $N=1000$. This shows SG method can reflect noise level in the condition of short data length. For the time series of state variable x in Logistic chaos system without noise interference, the symplectic geometry spectrums (see Fig. 25b) are slant in the beginning then turn into plane area with the increase of index i. In other words, the distribution of total energy on the different axes is obviously different and with increasing the embedding dimension, the slants of symplectic geometry spectrums transit into noise floor. So one can determine embedding dimension from the number of symplectic geometry spectrums over noise floor, in which its determining criterion is similar to that in [37]. From Fig. 25b, the embedding dimension of Logistic chaotic time series can be estimated at 4 because the symplectic geometry spectrums begin to turn into noise floor at index 5. In a similar way, for Lorenz chaos time series without noise, when sampling interval $\tau=0.005$, the embedding dimension can be estimated at 6 (see Fig. 25c).

Comparison of the results of our method (see Fig. 25b and 25c) and the results of SVD method (see Fig. 25d and 25e) shows that in SG method, the position of the noise floor is determined by the intrinsic dynamical structure of the nonlinear dynamic system rather than the numerical accuracy of the input data and the computation precision, but in SVD method, the noise floor was determined reversely[8, 37, 61].

In a word, the numerical experiments discuss that for the nonlinear dynamic systems, SG method can give the appropriate embedding dimension from their time series but SVD method cannot. So SG method is fit to deal with nonlinear systems.

3.7.4. Robustness of the embedding dimension estimation based on symplectic geometry

It is well known that the recent methods about embedding dimension are almost more or less subjective, or are affected by changes of the data length, noise, time lag, or sampling time, etc. Here, it is necessary that the robustness of the SG method is studied.

The effect of data length

In order to avoid the effect of the characteristics of the nonlinear system, this paper only considers and uses the noise to analyze the effect of data length. For Gauss white noise with mean value 0 and variance 1, when $N=1000$, the SG method can give better results than the SVD method (see Fig. 26a) because the total energy is distributed equably (see Fig. 25a).

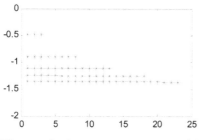

a. The symplectic geometry spectrums of Gauss white noise with mean value 0 and variance 1

b. The symplectic geometry spectrums of Logistic chaotic series with no noise

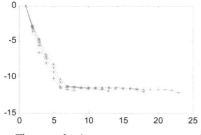

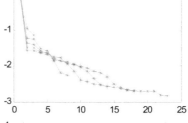

c. The symplectic geometry spectrums of Lorenz chaotic series with no noise, τ=0.005

d. The SVD principal components of Logistic chaotic series with no noise

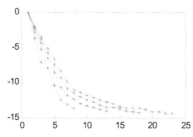

e. The SVD principal components of Lorenz chaotic series with no niose, τ=0.005

Figure 25. The study of embedding dimension based on symplectic geometry algorithm, N=1000, d=3, 8, 13, 18, 23, abscissa is d, ordinate is $\log(\mu_i / tr(\mu_i))$

And yet when N is rather large, e.g. N=10000, the SVD method can just have the similar results (see Fig. 26b) with Fig. 25a. These show that the SG method is more robust to changes of the data length than the SVD method. Then the SG method is fitter to the analysis of short time series.

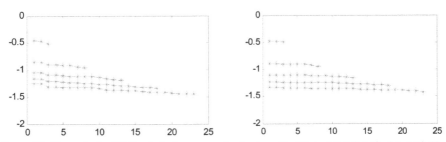

Figure 26. The analysis of SVD principal components of noise with different data length, d=3, 8, 13, 18, 23, abscissa is d, ordinate is $\log(\mu_i / tr(\mu_i))$

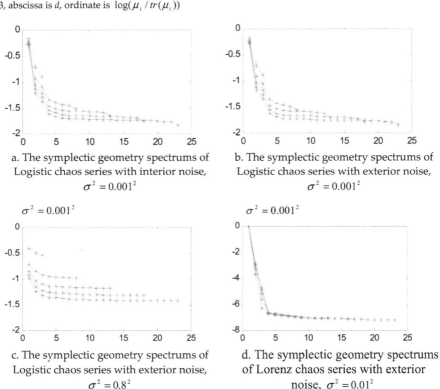

a. The symplectic geometry spectrums of
Logistic chaos series with interior noise,
$$\sigma^2 = 0.001^2$$

b. The symplectic geometry spectrums of
Logistic chaos series with exterior noise,
$$\sigma^2 = 0.001^2$$

c. The symplectic geometry spectrums of
Logistic chaos series with exterior noise,
$$\sigma^2 = 0.8^2$$

d. The symplectic geometry spectrums
of Lorenz chaos series with exterior
noise, $\sigma^2 = 0.01^2$

Figure 27. The study of symplectic geometry spectrum analysis in different noises, N=1000, d=3, 8, 13, 18, 23, abscissa is d, ordinate is $\log(\mu_i / tr(\mu_i))$

The effect of noise

At present, there are many estimators of appropriate embedding dimension, but it has gradually been realized that such estimators are useful only for low-dimensional noise-free systems; such systems, however, seem hardly to occur in the real life. Therefore, this paper studies the robustness of the SG method under noise. For the signal obtained from the real system, it is always contaminated by noise (inner noise or/and outer noise). Although contaminated by inner or/and outer noise, the embedding dimension of Logistic system can always be noted at 4 by using the SG method because the noise floor begins at the embedding dimension 5 (see Fig. 27a and 27b). These show either inner noise or outer noise has little impact on the symplectic geometry spectrums. On the further increase of noise, the position of noise floor is obviously raised from the Figure 27c, but the appropriate embedding dimension 2 can still be obtained. In the similar way, for Lorenz chaos time series without and with noise, when sampling interval τ=0.005, the embedding dimension is 6 without noise and 3 with noise, respectively (see Fig. 25c and Fig. 27d). These results show that the SG method is useful for Lorenz system with noise, too. Meanwhile, we find that the SG method can obtain the results similar to nonlinear high singular spectrum algorithm[62]. Thus, it further shows that the SG method can reflect intrinsic nonlinear characteristics of the raw data.

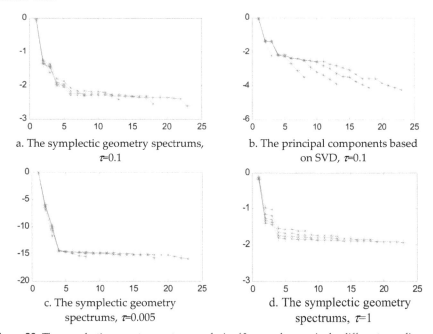

a. The symplectic geometry spectrums, τ=0.1

b. The principal components based on SVD, τ=0.1

c. The symplectic geometry spectrums, τ=0.005

d. The symplectic geometry spectrums, τ=1

Figure 28. The symplectic geometry spectrum analysis of Lorenz chaos series by different sampling intervals, N=1000, d=3, 8, 13, 18, 23, abscissa is d, ordinate is $\log(\mu_i / tr(\mu_i))$

The effect of sampling interval

For the changes of the sampling interval from τ=0.005 to τ=0.1, this paper finds that the embedding dimension can be estimated at 6 from the corresponding symplectic geometry spectrums of Lorenz chaos time series (see Fig. 25c and Fig. 28a), although the position of noise floor is constantly driven up. However, in the same condition, SVD method cannot give the appropriate embedding dimension (see Fig. 25e and 28b), the results of which are similar to the results of the literature[61]. Besides, no matter the sampling interval is over sampling or under sampling, SG method can always give the appropriate embedding dimension d of Lorenz chaos time series (see Fig. 28c and 28d) because the correlation dimension m of Lorenz system is 2.07, in general, if $d>m$, d is viable.

3.7.5. Analysis of the surface EMG signal based on symplectic geometry

For the action surface EMG signal (ASEMG) collected from a normal person, SVD method cannot give its appropriate embedding dimension (see Fig. 29a). The method based on correlation theory can do it but costs much time for computation. Here, SG method can fast obtain its embedding dimension. Figure 29b is the symplectic geometry spectrums of action surface EMG signal. The embedding dimension can be chosen as 6, which is the same as that of correlation dimension analysis[3]. This further shows that the SG method has stronger practicability for the small sets of experiment data.

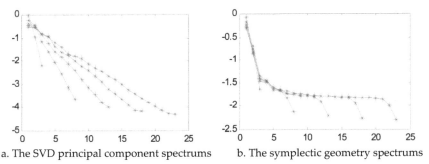

a. The SVD principal component spectrums   b. The symplectic geometry spectrums

Figure 29. The analysis of action surface EMG signal, d=3, 8, 13, 18, 23, abscissa is d, ordinate is $\log(\mu_i / tr(\mu_i))$

4. Study of nonlinear dynamical systems based on multifractal theory

Fractal is a kind of geometry structures that have similarity in structure, form or function between the local and the whole. In nature, almost every object is very complex and performs a self-organization phenomenon that is a spatiotemporal structure or state phenomenon by forming spontaneously. From the view of geometry structure, this object has its own self-similarity properties in many parts, called a multifractal system. This structure can often be characterized by a set of coefficients, such as multifractal dimension, wavelet multifractal energy dimension. The multifractal theory reflects the complexity and richness of the nature in essence.

4.1. Self-affine fractal[63-65]

Definition 1 Let the mapping $S: R^n \to R^n$. S is defined by

$$S(x) = T(x) + b \tag{69}$$

where T is a linear transformation on R^n. b is a vector in R^n. Thus, S is a combination of a translation, rotation, dilation and, perhaps, a reflection, called an affine mapping. Unlike similarities, affine mappings contract with differing ratios in different directions.

Theorem 1 Consider the iterated function system given by the contractions$\{S_1, \cdots, S_m\}$on $D \subset R^n$, so that

$$|S_i(x) - S_i(y)| \leq C_i|x - y|, \quad \forall x, y \in D \tag{70}$$

with $\exists C_i < 1$ for each i. Then there is a unique attractor F, i.e. a non-empty compact set such that

$$F = \bigcup_{i=1}^{m} S_i(F) \tag{71}$$

Moreover, if we define a transformation S on the class ϕ of non-empty compact sets by

$$S(E) = \bigcup_{i=1}^{m} S_i(E) \tag{72}$$

For $E \in \phi$, and write S^k for the kth iterate of S (so $S^0(E) = E$ and $S^k(E) = S(S^{k-1}(E))$ for $k \geq 1$), then

$$F = \bigcap_{k=1}^{\infty} S^k(E) \tag{73}$$

for every set $E \in \phi$ such that $S_i(E) \subset E$ for all i.

If an IFS consists of affine contractions $\{S_1, \cdots, S_m\}$ on R^n, the attractor F guaranteed by Theorem 1 is termed a self-affine set.

Since self-affine time series have a power-law dependence of the power-spectral density function on frequency, .self-affine time series exhibit long-range persistence. For a practical data, one can use the relationship of power spectrum and frequency to determine if the data has the self-affine fractal characteristic.

4.2. Spectrum analysis[65, 66]

Let a time series be $x(t)$, $t \in [0, T]$. Its spectrum is given by

$$X(f, T) = \int_0^T x(t) e^{2\pi i f t} dt \tag{74}$$

where f is frequency. The power spectrum of f is defined by

$$S(f) = \frac{1}{T}|X(f, T)|^2 \tag{75}$$

If the power spectrum obeys a power law

$$S(f) = K \cdot f^{-\beta} \tag{76}$$

for large f, the time series $x(t)$ has the self-affine fractal characteristic. The self-affine fractal dimension D is given

$$D = (5 - \beta)/2 \tag{77}$$

$S(f)$ is plotted as a function of f with log-log scaling. β is the negative of the slope of the best-fit straight line in the range of large f. Note that the value of β is a measure of the strength of persistence in a time series. $\beta > 1$ reflects strong persistence and nonstationary. $1 > \beta > 0$ describes weak persistence and stationary. $\beta = 0$ shows uncorrelated stationary. $\beta < 0$ indicates antipersistence and stationary. In all cases, however, a self-affine time series with a non-zero β has long-range (as well as short-range) persistence and anti-persistence. For small β, the correlations with large lag are small but are non-zero. This can be contrasted with time series that are not self-affine; these may have only short-range persistence (either strong or weak).

Although the self-affine mapping are varied in a continuous way, the dimension of the self-affine set need not change continuously. Unfortunately, the self-affine fractal situation is much more complicated. It is quite difficult to obtain a general formula for the dimension of self-affine sets. It is not enough that only one fractal dimension is used to describe the self-affine fractal time series. The multifractal dimensions have been proposed to describe this kind of the time series[67-72].

4.3. Multifractal dimension

For a measured time series of a multifractal system, its trajectory in phase space is often attracted to a bounded fractal object called strange attractor for which a whole set of dimension D_q has been introduced which generalize the concept of the Hausdorff dimension. Let X_1, ..., X_n be a point of the attractor in the phase space. The probability that the trajectory point is found within a ball of radius l around one of the inhomogeneously distributed points of the trajectory is denoted by

$$\mu(C_i) = \frac{1}{n} \sum_{i=1}^{n} \theta(l - \|X_i - X_j\|) \tag{78}$$

where $\theta(X)$ is the Heaviside step function. If $X \geq 0$, $\theta(X) = 1$; otherwise, $\theta(X) = 0$.

The q-order correlation integral is defined by

$$C_q(l) = \left(\frac{1}{n} \sum_{j=1}^{n} (\mu(C_i))^q \right)^{1/(q-1)} \tag{79}$$

The multifractal dimension D_q can be computed by the following equation:

$$D_q = \lim_{l \to 0} \frac{\ln(C_q(l))}{\ln(l)} = \begin{cases} \dfrac{1}{q-1} \lim_{l \to 0} \dfrac{\ln \sum\limits_{i=1}^{N(l)} [\mu(C_i)]^q}{\ln(l)} & q \neq 1 \\[4ex] \lim_{l \to 0} \dfrac{\sum\limits_{i=1}^{N(l)} \mu(C_i) \ln \mu(C_i)}{\ln(l)} & q = 1 \end{cases}$$
(80)

The above D_q is the multifractal dimension method based on Grassberger and Procaccia. The generalized correlation integral $C^q(l)$ which can be obtained from an experimental time series yields in a plot $\ln C^q(l)$ vs $\ln l$ straight lines with slopes D_q. For $q=0$, the D_0 is called the topological dimension, fractal dimension or capacity dimension. For $q=1$, the D_1 is called the information dimension. For $q=2$, the D_2 is called correlation dimension. The function D_q is monotonically decreasing with q and gives information about the inhomogeneity of the attractor. For simple fractals, called monofractals, such as a homogeneous attractor, the multifractal dimension D_q is constant. In the general case of multifractal objects, the values of D_q monotonically decrease as q increase[67]. The shape of the D_q can be considered a criterion confirming that the object is a nonuniform fractal. Furthermore, it can be determined if the object is a nonlinear, complex structure by using the multifractal dimension of the signal.

4.4. Analysis of surface EMG signal based on multifractal dimension

The surface EMG signal is a complicated physiological signal. Its distribution is clearly uneven (see Figure 30). When the surface EMG signal is studied by using the fractal method, one should first determine if the surface EMG signal is fractal. Then, its corresponding fractal dimension D can be estimated by Eq.(77) under a certain resolution. Figure 30 shows the self-affine fractal analysis of the surface EMG signals from Channel 1 during finger flexion, finger tension, forearm pronation and forearm supination (the results of Channel 2 are similar to those of Channel 1). It can be seen that the surface EMG signals have self-affine fractal characteristics. The results explain the physiological mechanism of the surface EMG signals.

In view of self-affine fractal characteristics, only one single fractal dimension is not easy to characterize the dynamics of surface EMG signals for different actions (see Table 4). There is little difference for the self-affine fractal dimensions of the four actions, where each type of action signals was chosen 100 sets of the data. The data length is 1000 points. In other words, it is difficult to identify the surface EMG signals of the different actions by using a single fractal dimension. The multifractal dimension values should be used to describe the action surface EMG signals during the arm movements.

	Finger flexion	Finger tension	Forearm pronation	Forearm supination
Channel 1	-0.2402±0.0725	-0.2571±0.0947	-0.0280±0.3250	0.0692±0.1418
Channel 2	0.0738±0.5734	-0.3199±0.2842	-0.0901±0.2591	-0.2343±0.2134

Table 4. The self-affine D of surface EMG signals during movements

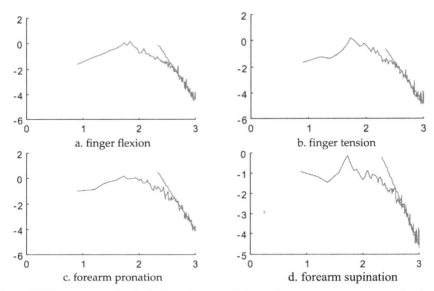

a. finger flexion   b. finger tension

c. forearm pronation   d. forearm supination

Figure 30. The analysis study of self-affine of surface EMG signal: Curve is power spectrum of surface EMG signal, line is straight line fit related part of curve; Abscissa is lg(f), ordinate is lg(Psd)

Here, we use the above multifractal dimension theory to analyze the action surface EMG signals. For the surface EMG signals of the four actions in channel 1, the multifractal analysis results are shown in Figure 31. The results of channel 2 are omitted since they are similar to those of channel 1. In the figure, the D_q-q curves are calculated under q =8, 7, 6, 5, 4, 3, 2, 1, 0, -1, -2, -3, -4, -5, -6, -7, -8. It can be seen that the D_q-q curves have a certain range. The results indicate that the surface EMG signals are non-uniform fractal structure signals. These are consistent with the results of the above self-affine fractal analysis. The parameter values with q can be used to classify the data. In theory, it will be more reasonable that multifractal dimensions are used to describe the surface EMG signals. However, the actual calculation process of the multifractal dimensions is very time-consuming. For the surface EMG signals, it is extremely difficult to meet the requirements of real-time classification.

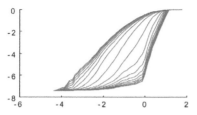

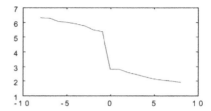

a. The multi-fractal curves of EMG signal during finger flexion; abscissa is ln(l), ordinate is ln($C_q(l)$)

b. The multi-fractal dimensions of curves in Fig. a; abscissa is q, ordinate is D_q

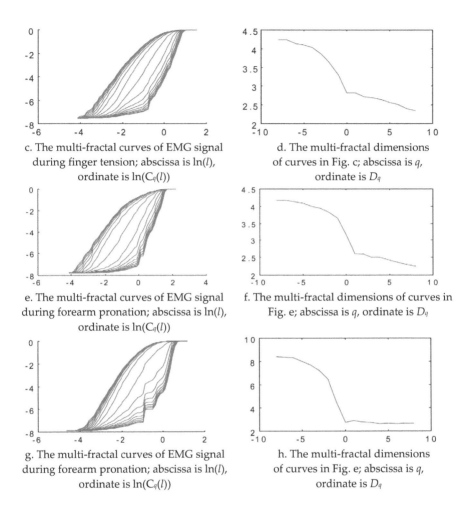

c. The multi-fractal curves of EMG signal during finger tension; abscissa is ln(l), ordinate is ln($C_q(l)$)

d. The multi-fractal dimensions of curves in Fig. c; abscissa is q, ordinate is D_q

e. The multi-fractal curves of EMG signal during forearm pronation; abscissa is ln(l), ordinate is ln($C_q(l)$)

f. The multi-fractal dimensions of curves in Fig. e; abscissa is q, ordinate is D_q

g. The multi-fractal curves of EMG signal during forearm pronation; abscissa is ln(l), ordinate is ln($C_q(l)$)

h. The multi-fractal dimensions of curves in Fig. e; abscissa is q, ordinate is D_q

Figure 31. The multi-fractal analysis of surface EMG signals during movements

5. Conclusion and future research

In order to investigate whether the essence of the surface EMG signal is stochastic or deterministic nonlinear (even chaotic), some emerging nonlinear time series analysis approaches are discussed in this chapter. These techniques are based on detecting and describing deterministic structure in the signal, such as surrogate data method, VWK model method, chaotic analysis method, symplectic geometry method, fractal analysis method, and so on.

The surrogate data method and VWK model mehtod are used to detect the surface EMG signal for arm movement and muscle fatigue. The results show that the surface EMG signal has deterministic nonlinear components. Moreover, our algorithm of surrogate data based on the null hypothesis 3 is proved that can completely satisfy the requirment of the null hypothesis 3. The VWK method with surrogate data can illuminate that not only the action but also fatigue surface EMG signals contain nonlinear dynamic properties.

Chaotic analysis techniques are reviewed and applied to investigate the surface EMG signals. The results show that the surface EMG signals have high-dimension chaotic dynamics by using correlation dimension and largest Lyapunov expoent techniques. For the estimation of embedding dimension, symplectic principal component analysis method is introduced and discussed. In comparison with correlation dimension algorithm and SVD analysis, symplectic geometry analysis is both very simple and reliable. The results show that symplectic geometry method is useful for determining of the system attractor from the experiment data.

The fractal theory is applied to study the fractal feature of the action surface EMG signal collected from forearm of normal person. The results show that he action surface EMG signal possesses the self-affine fractal characteristic. So, it is difficult to describe the surface EMG signals by using a single fractal dimension. The multifractal dimensions are used to analyze the action surface EMG signals during the arm movements. The results indicate that the surface EMG signals are non-uniform fractal structure signals. The multifractal dimension values can be used to identify the surface EMG signals for different movements.

For the nonlinear characteristics of the surface EMG signals, chaos and fractal theories will play the leading role in the nonlinear study of the surface EMG signals. The related methods need to be further researched and developed although these techniques have been applied to analyze the surface EMG signals. It provides a new way for the study of the quantitative analysis of physiology and pathology, sports medicine, clinical medical diagnostics and bionics of robot limb motion.

Apendix A

Theorem 1 proof:

$$
\begin{aligned}
\because \quad & J\begin{pmatrix} A & 0 \\ 0 & -A^* \end{pmatrix} J^{-1} \\
= & \begin{pmatrix} 0 & I_n \\ -I_n & 0 \end{pmatrix}\begin{pmatrix} A & 0 \\ 0 & -A^* \end{pmatrix}\begin{pmatrix} 0 & I_n \\ -I_n & 0 \end{pmatrix}^{-1} \\
= & \begin{pmatrix} -A^* & 0 \\ 0 & A \end{pmatrix} \\
= & -\begin{pmatrix} A & 0 \\ 0 & -A^* \end{pmatrix}^*
\end{aligned}
\tag{81}
$$

$\therefore$ According Definition 2, $\begin{pmatrix} A & 0 \\ 0 & -A^* \end{pmatrix}$ is a Hamilton matrix. $\square$

Theorem 2 proof:

Let S as a symplectic transform matrix, M as a Hamilton matrix. Then S^{-1} is also symplectic matrix. According Definition 1 and 2, there is

$$
\begin{aligned}
& J\left(SMS^{-1}\right)J^{-1} \\
& = JSJ^{-1}JMJ^{-1}JS^{-1}J^{-1} \\
& = S^{-*}\left(-M^*\right)S^* \\
& = -\left(SMS^{-1}\right)^*
\end{aligned}
$$
(82)

$\therefore SMS^{-1}$ is also a Hamilton matrix.

$$
\therefore SMS^{-1} \sim M
$$
(83)

So Hamilton matrix M keeps unchanged at symplectic similar transform. $\square$

Theorem 5 proof:

Let S_1, S_2,..., S_n as symplectic matrix, respectively. According Definition 1, there are

$$
\begin{aligned}
JS_1J^{-1} &= S_1^{-*} \\
JS_2J^{-1} &= S_2^{-*} \\
&\cdots \\
JS_nJ^{-1} &= S_n^{-*}
\end{aligned}
$$
(84)

$$
\begin{aligned}
& J\left(S_1S_2\cdots S_n\right)J^{-1} \\
& = JS_1J^{-1}JS_2J^{-1}J\cdots J^{-1}JS_nJ^{-1} \\
& = S_1^{-*}S_2^{-*}\cdots S_n^{-*} \\
& = \left(S_1S_2\cdots S_n\right)^{-*}
\end{aligned}
$$
(85)

So the product of sympletcic matrixes is also a symplectic matrix.

Theorem 6 proof:

In order to prove that H matrix is symplectic matrix, we only need to prove $H^*JH = J$.

$$
\begin{aligned}
H^*JH &= \begin{pmatrix} P & 0 \\ 0 & P \end{pmatrix}^* J \begin{pmatrix} P & 0 \\ 0 & P \end{pmatrix} \\
&= \begin{pmatrix} 0 & P^*P \\ -P^*P & 0 \end{pmatrix}
\end{aligned}
$$
(86)

$$\because P = I_n - \frac{2\varpi\varpi^*}{\varpi^*\varpi}$$

$$\therefore \quad P^* = P$$

$$P^*P = P^2$$

$$= \left(I_n - \frac{2\varpi\varpi^*}{\varpi^*\varpi} \right)\left(I_n - \frac{2\varpi\varpi^*}{\varpi^*\varpi} \right)$$

$$= I_n - \frac{4\varpi\varpi^*}{\varpi^*\varpi} + \frac{4\varpi(\varpi^*\varpi)\varpi^*}{(\varpi^*\varpi)(\varpi^*\varpi)} \tag{87}$$

$$= I_n$$

where $\varpi = (0,\cdots,0;\omega_k,\cdots,\omega_n)^T \neq 0$.

Plugging Eq.(87) into Eq.(86), we have:

$$H^*JH = J \tag{88}$$

$\therefore$ H is symplectic matrix.

$$H^*H = \begin{pmatrix} P & 0 \\ 0 & P \end{pmatrix}^* \begin{pmatrix} P & 0 \\ 0 & P \end{pmatrix}$$

$$= \begin{pmatrix} P^*P & 0 \\ 0 & P^*P \end{pmatrix} \tag{89}$$

$$= I_{2n}$$

$\therefore$ H is also unitary matrix.

$\therefore$ H is symplectic unitary matrix. $\square$

Apendix B

Theorem 7 suppose x and y are two unequal n dimension vectors, and $\|x\|_2 = \|y\|_2$, so there is elementary reflective array $H = 1 - 2\omega\omega^T$, which make $Hx = y$, where $\omega = \dfrac{x-y}{\|x-y\|_2}$.

It can be easily deduced from theorem 5, for non zero n dimension vector $x = (x_1, x_2, \cdots, x_n)^T$, notes $\alpha = \|x\|_2$, there is

$$Hx = \alpha e_1 \tag{90}$$

$$H = 1 - 2\varpi\varpi^T \tag{91}$$

$$e_1 = (1,0,\cdots,0)^T \tag{92}$$

$$\varpi = \frac{1}{\rho}(x - \alpha e_1) \tag{93}$$

$$\rho = \|x - \alpha e_1\|_2 \tag{94}$$

Then $\|\omega\|_2 = 1$, and H is elementary reflective array.

It's easy to testify, elementary reflective array H is symmetry matrix $(H^T = H)$, orthogonal matrix $(H^T H = 1)$ and involution matrix $(H^2 = 1)$.

For real symmetrical matrix A, Householder matrix H can be constructed as follows[73]. Notes A:

$$A = \begin{pmatrix} a_{11} & a_{12} & \cdots & a_{1n} \\ a_{21} & a_{22} & \cdots & a_{2n} \\ \vdots & \vdots & \cdots & \vdots \\ a_{n1} & a_{n2} & \cdots & a_{nn} \end{pmatrix} = \begin{pmatrix} a_{11} & A_{12}^{(1)} \\ \alpha_{21}^{(1)} & A_{22}^{(1)} \end{pmatrix} \tag{95}$$

First, suppose $\alpha_{21}^{(1)} \neq 0$, otherwise this column will be skipped and the next column will be considered until the ith column of $\alpha_{2i}^{(1)} \neq 0$. Set first column vector of A:

$$S^{(1)} = \left(a_{11}^{(1)}, a_{21}^{(1)}, \cdots, a_{n1}^{(1)}\right)^T = (a_{11}, a_{21}, \cdots, a_{n1}) \tag{96}$$

select elementary reflective array $H^{(1)}$:

$$H^{(1)} = I - 2\varpi^{(1)} (\varpi^{(1)})^T \tag{97}$$

where

$$\begin{cases} \alpha_1 = \|S^{(1)}\|_2 \\ E^{(1)} = (1, 0, \cdots, 0)^T \quad n \times 1 \\ \rho_1 = \|S^{(1)} - \alpha_1 E^{(1)}\| \\ \varpi^{(1)} = \frac{1}{\rho_1}\left(S^{(1)} - \alpha_1 E^{(1)}\right) \end{cases} \tag{98}$$

so, after $H^{(1)}$ transform, A is changed to a matrix with the first column is all zero except the first element is α_1, namely:

$$H^{(1)} A = \begin{pmatrix} \sigma_1 & a_{12}^{(2)} & \cdots & a_{1n}^{(2)} \\ 0 & a_{22}^{(2)} & \cdots & a_{2n}^{(2)} \\ \vdots & \vdots & \ddots & \vdots \\ 0 & a_{n2}^{(2)} & \cdots & a_{nn}^{(2)} \end{pmatrix} = A^{(2)} \tag{99}$$

Second, the same method is adopted to the second column vector of $A^{(2)}$, let

$$S^{(2)} = \left(0, a_{22}^{(2)}, \cdots, a_{n2}^{(2)}\right)^T \tag{100}$$

construct $H^{(2)}$ matrix :

$$H^{(2)} = I - 2\omega^{(2)} (\varpi^{(2)})^T \tag{101}$$

where,

$$\begin{cases} \alpha_2 = \left\| S^{(2)} \right\|_2 \\ E^{(2)} = (0,1,0,\cdots,0)^T \qquad n \times 1 \\ \rho_2 = \left\| S^{(2)} - \alpha_2 E^{(2)} \right\| \\ \varpi^{(2)} = \dfrac{1}{\rho_2} \left(S^{(2)} - \alpha_2 E^{(2)} \right) \end{cases} \qquad (102)$$

Using $H^{(2)}$, the second column of $A^{(2)}$ can be changed to all zero vector except the first and second elements, namely:

$$H^{(2)} A^{(2)} = A^{(3)} \qquad (103)$$

Householder matrix H can be obtained by repeating above mentioned method until $A^{(n)}$ becomes an upper triangle matrix:

$$H = H^{(n)} H^{(n-1)} \cdots H^{(1)} \qquad (104)$$

Author details

Min Lei and Guang Meng
Institute of Vibration, Shock and Noise, State Key Laboratory of Mechanical System and Vibration, Shanghai Jiao Tong University, Shanghai, P R China

Acknowledgement

This work was supported by the National Natural Science Foundation of China (No. 10872125 and No.69675002), Science Fund for Creative Research Groups of the National Natural Science Foundation of China(no. 50821003), State Key Lab of Mechanical System and Vibration , Project supported by the Research Fund of State Key Lab of MSV, China (Grant no. MSV-MS-2010-08) , Key Laboratory of Hand Reconstruction, Ministry of Health, Shanghai, People's Republic of China, Shanghai Key Laboratory of Peripheral Nerve and Microsurgery, Shanghai, People's Republic of China, Science and Technology Commission of Shanghai Municipality (no.06ZR14042). We also thank Chinese Academy of Engineering GU Yudong and Professor Zhang Kaili very much for providing related data and valuable discussions.

6. References

[1] J Theiler, S Eubank, A Longtin, et al., Testing for nonlinearity in time series: the method of surrogate data. Physica D, 1992. 58: 77-94.
[2] M Barahona and C-S Poon, Detection of nonlinear dynamics in short, noisy time series. Nature, 1996. 381: 215-217.
[3] M Lei, Z Z Wang, and Z J Feng, Detecting nonlinearity of action surface EMG signal. Phys. Lett. A, 2001. 290(5-6): 297-303.

[4] M Palus and D Hoyer, Detecting nonlinearity and phase synchronization with surrogate data. IEEE Engineering in Medical and Biology, 1998. 17(6): 40-45.

[5] C-S Poon and K M Christopher, Decrease of cardiac chaos in congestive heart failure. Nature, 1997. 389: 492-495.

[6] J Theiler and D Prichard, Constrained-realization Monte-Carlo method for hypothesis testing. Physica D, 1996. 94: 221-235.

[7] C S Poon and M Barahona, Titration of chaos with added noise. Proceedings of The National Academy of Sciences of The United States of America, 2001. 98(13): 7107-7112.

[8] J A Scheinkman and B LeBaron., Nonlinear dynamics and stock returns. Journal of Business, 1989. 62(3): 311-337.

[9] J L Breeden and N H Packard, Nonlinear analysis of data sampled nonuniformly in time. Physica D, 1992. 58(1-4): 273-283.

[10] A R Osborne and A Provenzale, Finite correlation dimension for stochastic systems with power-law spectra. Physica D, 1989. 35(3): 357-381.

[11] M Lei, Nonlinear Time Series Analysis and Its Applied Study in Surface EMG Signal. 2000, Shanghai Jiao Tong University (in chinese).

[12] T Schreiber and A Schmitz, Improved surrogate data for nonlinearity tests. Phys. Rev. Lett., 1996. 77(4): 635-638.

[13] M Lei and Z Z Wang, Application of surrogate data method in electromyograph analysis. Journal of Shanghai Jiao Tong University, 2000. 34(11): 1594-1597 (in Chinese).

[14] M Lei and Z Z Wang, Study of the surrogate data method for nonlinearity of time series. Journal of Electronics and Information Technology, 2001. 23(3): 248-254 (in Chinese).

[15] M Lei, Z J Feng, and Z Z Wang, The Volterra-Wiener-Korenberg model nonlinear test method. Journal of Shanghai Jiao Tong University, 2003. 37(2): 269-272 (in Chinese).

[16] M Lei and G Meng, The influence of noise on nonlinear time series detection based on Volterra-Wiener-Korenberg model. Chaos, Solitons and Fractals, 2008. 36: 512-516.

[17] E N Lorenz, Determinstic nonperiodic flow. Journal of The Atmospheric Sciences, 1963. 20: 130-141.

[18] T Y Li and J A Yorke, Period three implies chaos. Amer Math Monthly, 1975. 82: 985-992.

[19] R M May, Simple mathematical models with very complicated dynamics. Nature, 1976. 261: 459-467.

[20] G U Yule., On a method of investigating periodicities in disturbed series with special reference to wolfer's sunspot numbers. Phil. Trans. R. Soc. London A, 1927. 226(636-646): 267-298

[21] F Takens, Detecting Strange Attractors in Turbulence. Dynamical Systems and Turbulence, 1980. 898: p. 366-381.

[22] N H Packard, J P Crutchfield, J D Farmer, et al., Geometry from a time series. Phys. Rev. Lett., 1980. 45: 712-716.

[23] K Vibe and J M Vesin, On chaos detection methods. International Journal of Bifurcation and Chaos, 1996. 6(3): 529-543.

[24] A M Fraser, Information and entropy in strange attractors. IEEE Trans. Inf. Theory, 1989. 35(2): 245-262.

[25] B Cheng and H Tong, Orthoggonal Projection, Embeding Dimension and Sample size in chaotic times series from a statistical perspective. Nonlinear time series and chaos, 1994. 2(15): 1-30.

[26] H S Kim, R Eykholt, and J D Salas, Nonlinear dynamics, delay times, and embedding windows. Physica D, 1999. 127: 48-60.

[27] D Kugiumtzis, State space reconstruction parameters in the analysis of chaotic time series — the role of the time window length. Physica D, 1996. 95(1): 13–28.

[28] M T Rosenstein, J J Collins, and C J D Luca, Reconstruction expansion as a geometry-based framework for choosing proper delay times. Physica D, 1994. 73: 82-98.

[29] J M Martinerie, A M Albano, A I Mees, et al., Mutual information, strange attractors, and the optimal estimation of dimension. Phys. Rev. A 1992. 45: 7058-7064.

[30] A M Fraser and H L Swinney, Independent coordinates for strange attractors from mutual information. Phys. Rev. A, 1986. 33(2): 1134-1140.

[31] D S Broomhead and G P King, Extracting qualitative dynamics from experimental data. Physica D, 1986. 20(2-3): 217–236.

[32] M Knennel, R Brown, and H Abarbanel., Determining embedding dimension for phase — space reconstruction using a geometrical construction. Phys. Rev. A, 1992. 45: 3403–3411.

[33] P Grassberger and I Procaccia, Measuring the strangeness of strange attractors. Physica D, 1983. 9(1-2): 189-208.

[34] A Galka, T Maaß, and P G., Estimating the dimension of high-dimensional attractors: a comparison between two algorithms. Physica D, 1998. 121: 237-251.

[35] K Judd and A Mees, Embedding as a modeling problem. Physica D, 1998. 120: 273-286.

[36] L Cao, Practical method for determining the minimum embedding dimension of a scalar time series. Physica D, 1997. 110(1-2): 43–50.

[37] M Palus and I Dvorak, Singular-value decomposition in attractor reconstruction: pitfalls and precautions. Physica D, 1992. 55: 221-234.

[38] K Judd, An improved estimator of dimension and some comments on providing confidence intervals. Physica D, 1992. 56: 216-228.

[39] P Grassberger, Generalized dimensions of strange attractors. Phys. Lett. A, 1983. 97: 227-234.

[40] P Grassberger and I Procaccia, Characterization of strange attractors. Phys. Rev. Lett., 1983. 50: 346–349.

[41] M Ding, C Grebogi, E Ott, et al., Plateau onset for correlation dimension: when does it occur? Phys. Rev. Lett. , 1993. 70: 3872–3875.

[42] M Small and K Judd, Detecting nonlinearity in experimental data. International Journal of Bifurcation and Chaos, 1998. 8(6): 1231-1244.

[43] A Wolf, J Swift, H Swinney, et al., Determining Lyapunov exponents from a time series. Physica D, 1985. 16: 285-317.

[44] M Sano and Y Sawada, Measurement of the Lyapunov spectrum from a chaotic time series. Phys. Rev. Lett., 1985. 55(10): 1082-1085.

[45] M T Rosenstein, J J Collins, and C J D Luca, A practical method for calculating largest lyapunov exponents from small data sets. Physica D, 1993. 65: 117-134.

[46] A I Mees, P E Rapp, and L S Jennings, Singular-value decomposition and embedding dimension. Phys. Rev. A, 1987. 36: 340–346.

[47] A M Fraser., Reconstructing attractors from scalar time series : a comparison of singular system and redundancy criteria. Physica D, 1989. 34: 391-404.

[48] A Brandsttater, H L Swinney, and G I Chapman, Characterizing turbulent channel flow. in: Dimensions and entropies in chaotic systems, G. Mayer-Kree(Ed.), Springer, Berlin 1986: 150.

[49] M Lei, Z Z Wang, and Z J Feng, A method of embedding dimension estimation based on symplectic geometry. Phys. Lett. A, 2002. 303(2-3): 179-189.

[50] X Lu and R Schmid, Symplectic integration of Sine-Gordon type systems. Mathematics and Computers in Simulation, 1999. 50: 255-263.

[51] Z G Ying and W Q Zhu, Exact stationary solutions of stochastically excited and dissipated gyroscopic systems. International Journal of Non-Linear Mechanics, 2000. 35: 837-848.

[52] A C J Luo and R P S Han, The resonance theory for stochastic layers in nonlinear dynamic systems. Chaos, Solitons and Fractals, 2001. 12: 2493-2508.

[53] K Feng, Proceeding of the 1984 Beijing Symposium on Differential Geometry and Differential Equations: Computation of partial differential equations, ed. F. Kang. 1985: Science Press, 42.

[54] C V Loan, A Symplectic Method for Approximating All the Elgenvalues of a Hamiltonian Matrix. Linear Algebra and Its Applications, 1984. 61: 233-251.

[55] M Lei, Z Z Wang, and Z J Feng, The application of symplectic geometry on nonlinear dynamics analysis of the experimental data. 14th International Conference on Digital Signal Processing Proceeding, 2002. 1-2: 1137-1140.

[56] M Lei and G Meng, Detecting nonlinearity of sunspot number. International Journal of Nonlinear Sciences and Numerical Simulation, 2004. 5(4): 321-326.

[57] X Niu, F Qu, and N Wang, Evaluating Sprinters' Surface EMG Signals Based on EMD and Symplectic Geometry. J of Ocean Univ. of Qingdao, 2005. 35(1): 125-129.(in Chinese).

[58] H Xie, Z Z Wang, and H Huang, Identification determinism in time series based on symplectic geometry spectra. Phys. Lett. A, 2005. 342(1-2): 156-161.

[59] M Lei and G Meng, Symplectic principal component analysis: a new method for time series analysis. Mathematical Problems in Engineering, 2011. 2011: Article ID 793429, 14pages.

[60] M Lei and G Meng, A noise reduction method for continuous chaotic systems based on symplectic geometry. The Seventh International Conference on Vibration Engineering and Technology of Machinery, 2011. 1: Article ID 173, 6pages.

[61] Y Gong and J Xu, Chaos signal and noise. Signal Processing, 1997. 13(2): 112-118 (in Chinese)

[62] J Yuan and X C Xiao, Higher-order singular-spectrum analysis of nonlinear time series. Acta Physica Sinica, 1998. 47(6): 897-905 (in Chinese).

[63] B B Mandelbrot, Self-affine fractals and fractal dimension. Physica Scripta, 1985. 32: 257-260.

[64] B B Mandelbrot, The fractal geometry of Nature. 1982: San Francisco: Freeman.

[65] K Falconer, Fractal Geometry: Mathematical Foundations and Applications. 2003: John Wiley &Sons Ltd. 337.

[66] B D Malamud and D L Turcotte, Self-affine time series: measures of weak and strong persistence. Journal of Statistical Planning and Inference, 1999. 80: 173-196.

[67] A N Pavlov and V S Anishchenko, Multifractal analysis of complex signals. Physics-Uspekhi, 2007. 50(8): 819-834.

[68] R H Riedi, M S Crouse, V J Ribeiro, et al., A multifractal wavelet model with application to network traffic. IEEE Trans. On Information Theory, 1999. 45(3): 992-1018.

[69] A Z R Langi, K Soemintapura, and W Kinsner. Multifractal processing of speech signals. in International Conference on Information, Communications and Signal Processing. 1997.

[70] Z Xu and S Xiao. Fractal dimension of surface EMG and its determinants. in Proceedings of the 19th Annual International Conference of the IEEE Engineerings in Medicine and Biology Society. 1997.

[71] O Adeyemi and G F Boudreaux-Bartels. Improved accuracy in the singularity spectrum of multifractal chaotic time series. in IEEE International Conference on Acoustics, Speech, and Signal Processing. 1997.

[72] C J Aumuth, Fractals dimension of electromyographic signals recorded with surface electrodes during isometric contractions with muscle activation. Muscle & Nerve, 1994. 17: 953-954.

[73] J Huang, The practical modeling method of static and dynamic mathematical model. 1988, Beijing: Mechanical Industry Press (in Chinese).

Chapter 3

EMG Decomposition and Artefact Removal

Adriano O. Andrade, Alcimar B. Soares,
Slawomir J. Nasuto and Peter J. Kyberd

Additional information is available at the end of the chapter

1. Introduction

Traditionally, in clinical electromyography (EMG), neurophysiologists assess the state of the muscle by studying basic units of an EMG signal, which are referred to as motor unit action potentials (MUAPs). Information regarding the morphology and rate of occurrence of MUAPs is often used for diagnosis of neuromuscular disorders. In addition, recent studies have shown that the analysis of the energy content of MUAPs is a possible way for discriminating among normal, neurogenic, and myopathic MUAPs [38], illustrating, thus, the clinical value of the interpretation of MUAP information.

A common way of obtaining such information is by observing MUAP activities on an oscilloscope and listening to their audio characteristics over the speakers. When doing this, the researcher is implicitly performing a time and frequency analysis of MUAPs. However, the results of this analysis are dependent on the experience of the investigator and on his ability to extract relevant information from the visual and auditory analysis. Furthermore, this procedure is time-consuming and prone to error.

The drawbacks related to the procedure described above have motivated the use of computer-based techniques for extraction of MUAPs from EMG signals [3, 19, 22, 27, 29, 32, 40]. Such methods, also known as EMG decomposition techniques, aim at classifying MUAPs generated by a common source into the same group. The results of this classification may provide information regarding the orchestration of the neuromuscular system, and therefore of the state of the muscle. A similar problem, often referred to as spike sorting, is found in the study of neuronal activities [25]. In this case, neuronal action potentials from the same source are classified into a common group.

Originally, the investigation of MUAP activities belonged to needle electromyographic (NEMG) studies, mainly because surface electrodes may easily produce an integration of many potentials, which precludes accurate study of their individual form. However, some recent studies have shown that the use of surface electrodes may be successfully applied for detection of MUAPs from superficial muscles [8]. This advancement has received widespread support among researchers and clinicians because of the ease of use, reduced risk of infection, and the greater number of motor unit action potential trains obtained compared to needle sensor techniques [47].

Currently, computer-based EMG has become an indispensable tool for investigations seeking to explain the state of the muscle. Different methodologies, ranging from simple quantitative measures to automatic systems that enable the assessment of neuromuscular disorders, have been developed [30]. Such tools are important for standardization of results and also they may reveal important features in the signals, which might be barely perceived from a manual analysis [35].

A typical system for extraction of MUAPs from EMG signals may require several stages of signal processing, for instance, signal detection and filtering (i.e., artefact removal) [45], feature extraction or selection [36], data clustering or classification [23]. Specific research may be carried out in each of these steps.

2. Strategies for EMG decomposition

One of the most rudimentary strategies for isolation of MUAPs belonging to a common group is by means of a thresholding scheme. The central idea of this technique is to use a voltage threshold trigger for detection of MUAPs that have similar height, which is represented by the amplitude of the highest peak of a MUAP. In this method the experimenter positions the recording electrode so that MUAPs of interest are maximally separated from the background activity (noise). MUAP activities are then measured with a hardware threshold trigger, which generates a pulse whenever the measured voltage crosses the threshold. Such pulses may be used for triggering data collection and further storage of MUAPs or their occurrence time in a computer. The main advantages of this method are that: (i) It is easy to apply since it requires minimal hardware and software; (ii) It is a good starting point for detection of the strongest MUAPs. The main drawbacks of this technique are that: (i) The threshold level, mainly dependent on the signal-to-noise ratio, determines the trade-off between missed spikes (false negatives) and the number of background events that cross the threshold (false positives); (ii) Only a single feature (the MUAP highest peak) is used for data classification. As a consequence of this strategy two MUAPs with different shapes might be grouped together because they have similar peak amplitude.

The drawbacks related to the technique discussed above highlight the importance of a pre-processing stage prior to grouping MUAPs. The presence of high levels of background activity in the signal suggests that the use of a filter for reduction of the background activity is necessary. Different digital filters may be used for this purpose. Typically high band-pass filters are used for attenuation of very low frequency components in the signal related to noise, which can be either inherent from the hardware used for data acquisition or the contribution of distant MUAPs from the detection point.

Another common approach is the use of differential filters. Such filters are low-pass filters and have been used in many investigations. The main drawback of such filters is that they may generate artificial spikes and modify the shape of MUAPs. This has motivated the use of alternative filtering procedures, for instance, wavelets and a spatial filter, known as a Laplacian filter. The implementation of these filters as well as the introduction of an alternative method for EMG signal filtering is further discussed in the chapter.

Another relevant pre-processing step is the one that segments the EMG signal into windows containing active and inactive segments. This is a signal detection stage which aims to identify the activities of single MUAPs or their combinations, which is known as MUAP overlaps. Furthermore, this step separates noise in inactive segments from useful information in active segments. The detection of active and inactive segments may be performed visually or manually, i.e. the researcher may classify regions of an electromyographic signal into one of those categories, however such a method is time-consuming and requires concentration, which may introduce inconsistency in the signal analysis.

Different approaches may be employed for automation of this pre-processing stage: (i) The use of the root-mean square of the EMG signal together with a pre-defined threshold; (ii) A threshold proportional to the maximum peak in the signal; (iii) A threshold which is manually adjusted; (iv) Wavelets. The main assumption of this method is that there might be similarity between the mother wavelet and action potentials, and when the correlation between an active window and the mother wavelet is high an active segment is detected.

As one may note there exists a variety of strategies that could be considered for automation of the detection of active and inactive segments. Techniques that make an assumption about a pre-defined height and width of MUAPs may be more susceptible to failures, i.e. active regions that do not fit the predefined window will not be detected. Note also that the level of the background activity in the signal will also influence the determination of the beginning and end of active segments. The detection of active regions is further discussed in this chapter.

After detection of active regions it is possible to group them into logical units (clusters), however, it is very common to obtain features from those regions prior to data clustering. For example, morphological features of MUAPs, i.e. duration, amplitude, area, number of phases (number of baseline crossings) and number of turns (number of positive and negative peaks) have been employed. Other successful approaches include the use of coefficients of the Fourier transform, the coefficients of the Wavelet transform, the use of time samples of the band-pass filtered signal and low-pass differentiated signal, and the use of autoregressive and cepstral coefficients. Some other approaches, known as feature extraction and selection procedures, try to obtain features that maximize cluster separability. Examples of the use of such techniques include the application of Principal Component Analysis (PCA) and Independent Component Analysis (ICA).

The grouping of MUAPs is commonly performed by means of at least three distinct strategies: (i) Template matching: raw MUAPs, referred to as MUAP templates, are first classified or identified, and then used for classification of new MUAPs. The initial MUAP templates may be manually selected from the EMG signal or be chosen automatically from a clustering procedure. During data classification, usually MUAP templates are modified by an update rule, which takes into account the variability of MUAP shapes in the data set; (ii) Clustering: a clustering technique is used for grouping patterns represented by features selected from active regions; (iii) Hybrid: in this approach, first a clustering technique is used for grouping part of the data set (normally the first 3 to 5 seconds), and then the non-classified data set is grouped into one of the classes defined in the first step.

Both the template matching and hybrid techniques require a priori identification of patterns in the data set before classification of the entire data set. The main disadvantage of these methods is that if new MUAP classes appear they will not be identified. The main advantage is that extra information regarding MUAP activities, e.g. the study of the firing time of MUAPs, may be taken into account in the final classification. The clustering approach has the advantage that it makes no assumptions about the data set to be grouped.

The main processing steps discussed so far form the basis of a complete EMG decomposition system. When the final application of such system is to study the firing behaviour of sources that generate MUAPs, it may be necessary to include an extra stage that deals with a problem known as MUAP overlaps. Overlapping spikes occur when two or more spikes fire simultaneously. When using the clustering technique for grouping active segments it may be possible to detect such overlaps as outliers. There are at least three strategies for dealing with overlaps: (i) Once a spike is classified it is subtracted from the active segment, in the hope that this will improve the classification of subsequent spikes. This approach requires a template of the spike. It yields reasonable results when two spikes are separated well enough so that the first can be accurately classified, but fails when the spikes are close together. Another problem with this approach is that the subtraction can introduce more noise into the waveform if the spike model (template) is not accurate. Also subtraction-based approaches may introduce spurious spike-like shapes if the spike occurrence is not accurately estimated; (ii) Another approach is to compare all possible combinations of two or more spike models. However, for some applications the computation time for performing this comparison may be prohibitive; (iii) The use of multiple electrodes or an array of electrodes may reduce the problem of overlapping spikes, because what appears as an overlap on one channel might be an isolated unit on another. Since the main aim of solving the overlapping problem is to increase the accuracy of estimators (e.g. mean) obtained from the firing of motor units, an alternative option might be to work directly with a precise estimate of the estimator considering missing data points (i.e that some MUAPs are missing).

Finally, once the system is designed and implemented it is important to test its accuracy. At least three methods are well accepted for this purpose: (i) Synthetic signals: artificial EMG signals are generated and employed for testing the stages of the system. The main advantage of this approach is that the characteristics of the analyzed signal are totally known; (ii) Manual classification of MUAPs: MUAPs are visually classified by the researcher and the results of this classification are used as reference for evaluation of the automatic classification; (iii) Comparison between MUAP activities from different channels: the consistency of the decomposition data of the same units from two different electrodes provides an indirect measure of the accuracy in real data decomposition.

3. Artefact removal from EMG signals

The detection of electromyographic signals is a very complex process, which is affected not only by the muscle anatomy and the physiological process responsible for the signal generation but also by external factors, for instance, the inherent noise of the hardware employed in the signal amplification and digitalization. As a result EMG signals are often corrupted by noise.

It may be very difficult, if possible at all, to extract useful information from very poor signal-to-noise ratio EMG signals. In some applications, for example, the decomposition of electromyographic signals, a high level of background activity could impede the accurate segmentation of the signal into regions of activity that may represent the activity of single motor unit action potentials, influencing thus the final results of the EMG decomposition.

3.1. Conventional methods for EMG signal noise removal

3.1.1. Low-pass differential filter

Since its introduction, the low-pass differential filter (LPD) [44] has been widely employed in EMG signal processing [15, 19, 32, 40–42]. This filter is implemented in the time-domain as:

$$y_k = \sum_{n=1}^{N} (x_{k+n} - x_{k-n}), \tag{1}$$

where x_k is the discrete input time-series and y_k is the filtered output. N is the window width to adjust the cut-off frequency. Increasing N will reduce the cut-off frequency of the filter. This may be easily perceived if Equation 1 is studied in the frequency domain.

For this, consider the following difference equation obtained from Equation 1:

$$y[k] = \sum_{n=1}^{N} x[k+n] - \sum_{n=1}^{N} x[k-n]. \tag{2}$$

Its representation in the frequency domain may be obtained via its Z transform as follows,

$$Z(y[k]) = Z \left(\sum_{n=1}^{N} x[k+n] \right) - Z \left(\sum_{n=1}^{N} x[k-n] \right)$$

$$Z(y[k]) = \sum_{n=1}^{N} Z(x[k+n]) - \sum_{n=1}^{N} Z(x[k-n])$$

$$Z(y[k]) = Y(z) = \sum_{n=1}^{N} z^n X(z) - \sum_{n=1}^{N} z^{-n} X(z)$$

$$Y(z) = X(z) \left(\sum_{n=1}^{N} (z^n - z^{-n}) \right) \Bigg|_{z=e^{\frac{j2\pi f}{f_{sr}}}}$$

where the ratio $Y(z)/X(z)$ is the filter transfer function $H(z)$, f is the frequency in Hz and f_{sr} is the sampling frequency in Hz.

Figure 1 presents the results of the estimate of the filter transfer function with different sizes of windows, $N = 40$ and $N = 20$. Note how the cut-off frequency is shifted to a higher frequency when the window size is reduced.

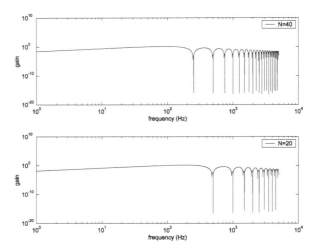

Figure 1. Frequency response of an LPD filter with window width 20 and 40.

The main advantages of using the LPD filter are that it is very easy to implement, and it is considerably fast for real-time applications, but some drawbacks regarding this filter are discussed in [46]:

- Under conditions of low signal-to-noise ratio the relatively strong high frequency noise (background activity) may be accentuated;
- Since the LPD filter is not an ideal low-pass filter, there will exist severe Gibbs phenomenon, that is, the leakage of energy frequency out of the filter pass-band as illustrated in the Bode diagrams shown in Figure 1. As a result, many high frequency noise components will pass through the filter.

3.1.2. Weighted low-pass differential filter

The weighted low-pass differential filter (WLPD) was proposed in [46] as an alternative to the LPD filter. The main difference is that an appropriately weighted window is included in Equation 2 for reduction of the Gibbs effect. The WLPD filter is implemented in the time-domain as:

$$y_k = \sum_{n=1}^{N} w(n)(x_{k+n} - x_{k-n}),$$

(3)

where $w(n)$ is an N point windowing function. Several windows such as Barlett, Hamming and Hanning may be employed. If a rectangular window is used then Equation 3 is an LPD filter. Similarly to the LPD filter the WLPD is very easy to implement and considerably fast for real-time applications, but results presented in [17, 46] show that phase distortion may

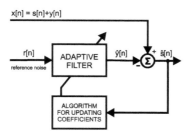

Figure 2. Adaptive noise canceller. $x[n]$ is the noise corrupted signal, $s[n]$ is the noise free signal, $y[n]$ the noise and $r[n]$ the reference noise. $\hat{y}[n]$ is the estimated noise, whereas $\hat{s}[n]$ the estimated signal.

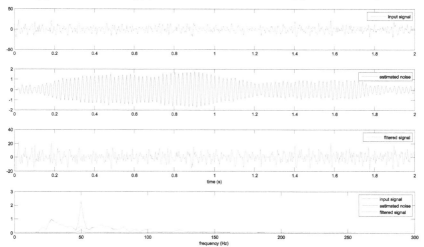

Figure 3. Example of application of the adaptive noise cancelling on a sample of EMG signal. The corrupted signal (top) is contrasted with the cleaned signal. The power spectra of the signals are shown at the bottom and illustrate the effect of the application of the filter on the 50 Hz component.

be present in the filtered signal and depending on the level of noise false spikes may be generated.

3.1.3. Adaptive 50/60 Hz noise cancellation

When the source of noise is well known it is possible to employ methods for adaptively reduce its influence over the desired signal. This is, for instance, the aim of adaptive 50/60 Hz noise cancellation based on the least mean square (LMS) algorithm [2].

The block diagram shown in Figure 2 depicts the main idea of the adaptive noise cancelling algorithm. The signal $s[n]$ is corrupted by the noise $y[n]$ yielding the corrupted signal $x[n]$. The adaptive algorithm will estimate parameters for a filter capable of attenuating the desired components and maintaining relevant information from the signal. The piece of code below is a Matlab function created for attenuating 50 Hz noise from signals. It was used to illustrate the application of the technique on an EMG signal which was strongly corrupted by 50 Hz noise. The plots given in Figure 3 show the input signal, the estimated noise and the filtered signal. The power spectra of these signals are given in the graph at the bottom. Their analysis allows us to conclude that the application of the adaptive filter attenuated the undesired 50 Hz component. Note that the 50 Hz component is also part of the EMG signal, therefore its complete elimination is not desired.

```
function [EstimatedNoise,filteredSig50Hz] = NoiseRemoval(x,fs)
%% Function name....: NoiseRemoval
% Description......:
%                    This function estimates a filtered signal based on a
%                    50Hz noise optimal filter (LMS algorithm)
% Parameters.......:
%                    x ......-> input time-series
%                    fs......-> sampling frequency (Hz)
% Return...........:
%                    EstimatedNoise... -> estimated 50 Hz noise
%                    filteredSig50Hz.. -> filtered signal (50 Hz noise free signal)

mu = 0.001; %constant of convergence of the LMS algorithm
taps = 10; %filter order
t = [0:1:length(x)-1]/fs;
d = sin(2*pi*t*50);  % reference noise (component to be removed from the input signal)
ha = adaptfilt.lms(taps,mu);
[y,e] = filter(ha,d,y);
[EstimatedNoise,filteredSig50Hz] = filter(ha,d,e);
```

3.1.4. Signal filtering based on wavelets

One of the main applications of wavelets is noise removal from corrupted signals. A general procedure for signal de-noising involves the following three steps that have been successfully applied [14, 16, 33]:

1. Signal decomposition;
2. Detail coefficients thresholding;
3. Signal reconstruction.

In the first step, both a wavelet prototype and the decomposition level (N) are chosen, and the wavelet decomposition of the signal at level N is performed. In the next step, for each level from 1 to N, a threshold, t_N, is selected and soft-thresholding is applied to detail coefficients as shown in Equation 4.

$$Y_N = sign(D_N)(|D_N| - t_N)_+ \qquad (4)$$

where Y_N is the de-noised version of the Nth detail coefficients and the function $(x)_+$ is defined as

$$(x)_+ = \begin{cases} 0, & x < 0 \\ x, & x >= 0. \end{cases} \qquad (5)$$

Finally, in the third step the denoised signal is estimated by using the original approximation coefficients of level N and the modified detail coefficients of levels from 1 to N. The application of this procedure is illustrated in the following example.

3.1.5. Example of application

The procedure for noise removal based on wavelets is applied to an experimental surface EMG signal in this section. The main aim is to attenuate the background activity present in the signal and at the same time to preserve its shape.

The Matlab Wavelet Toolbox[1] is used for data processing (see Figure 4). The EMG signal is decomposed into three levels ($N = 5$) and the $db5$ wavelet prototype is employed. The choice for the decomposition level may be justified by the fact that this signal is mostly contaminated by high frequency noise that will be highlighted by short time-scale components (e.g. detail coefficients of the first and second level) and therefore further decomposition would not contribute significantly to the final form of the filtered signal. The criteria for selection of the wavelet family (Daubechies) is mainly because of its reported success in removing/attenuating noise from EMG signals, and in its use for feature extraction from MUAPs [18, 37, 48].

The results of the signal decomposition are depicted in Figure 4. A window of the input EMG signal together with its filtered version are presented in Figure 5.

3.2. EMG signal filtering based on Empirical Mode Decomposition

In this section a novel algorithm for signal de-noising based on the Empirical Mode Decomposition (EMD) method is presented [7]. The developed filter may be employed as an alternative to the approach based on wavelets described above.

3.2.1. The Empirical Mode Decomposition method

Huang et al. (1998) [21] described a new technique for analyzing nonlinear and non-stationary data. The key part of the method is the Empirical Mode Decomposition (EMD) method, in which any complicated data set can be adaptively decomposed into a finite, and often small, number of Intrinsic Mode Functions (IMFs). The name Intrinsic Mode Function is adopted because those components represent the oscillation modes embedded in the data. In the case of Fourier analysis, oscillation modes (i.e. components) in a signal are defined in terms of sine and cosine waves. The EMD thus defines oscillation modes in terms of IMFs, which are functions that satisfy two conditions [21]:

1. In the whole time-series, the number of extrema and the number of zero crossings must be either equal or differ at most by one. Note that extrema are either local minima or local maxima. Furthermore, a sample g_i in a time-series is a local maximum if $g_i > g_{i-1}$ and $g_i > g_{i+1}$, and a sample q_i is a local minimum if $q_i < q_{i-1}$ and $q_i < q_{i+1}$, where i is a discrete time.

---

[1] This toolbox can be invoked by typing *wavemenu* in the Matlab command environment.

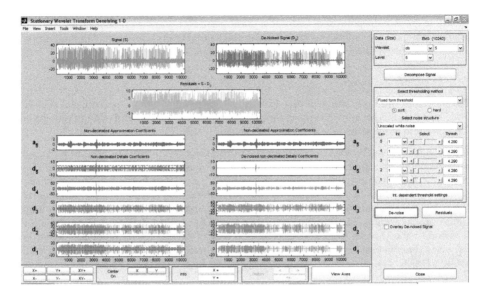

Figure 4. Graphical user interface of the Wavelet Matlab Toolbox used for signal denoising. The EMG signal and its denoised version are shown. The wavelet components are individually denoised by using a thresholding scheme.

2. At any point in the time-series, the mean value of the envelopes, one defined by the local maxima (upper envelope) and the other by the local minima (lower envelope), is zero.

The definition above is empirical and currently there is no explicit equation for estimating IMFs, thus any arbitrary time-series that satisfies conditions 1 and 2 is an IMF. Furthermore, by means of the analysis of the power spectra of IMFs it is possible to verify that these functions represent the original signal decomposed into different time-scales (or frequency bandwidths). This is illustrated in [4, 6]. Thus, both wavelets and the Empirical Mode Decomposition provide the decomposition of a signal into different time-scales. The main difference is that one method performs the signal decomposition adaptively and based solely on the available data, whereas the other normally uses a set of pre-fixed filters.

3.2.2. The algorithm for signal filtering based on the EMD

The success of the general procedure for noise removal using wavelets is based on the fact that it is possible to filter signal components individually instead of filtering the original signal. This is desirable because some components may highlight the noise and thus it may be easier to attenuate its presence.

Similarly, the Empirical Mode Decomposition also provides the decomposition of a signal into different time-scales or IMFs. This means that it is also possible to filter signal components individually instead of the original signal. This suggests that the strategy for signal de-noising

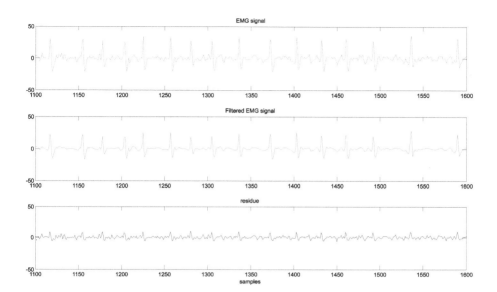

Figure 5. Segment of the EMG signal shown in Figure 4. The filtered signal and the residue is also presented.

based on wavelets may also be applied to intrinsic mode functions. Thus the following procedure was proposed for EMG signal filtering [3, 7]:

1. Decompose the signal into IMFs;
2. Threshold the estimated IMFs;
3. Reconstruct the signal.

This procedure is practical, mainly due to the empirical nature of the EMD method, and it may be applied to any signal as the EMD does not make any assumption about the input time-series. A block diagram describing the steps for its application is shown in Figure 6. First, the EMD method is used for decomposing the input signal into intrinsic mode functions, $IMF_1, \ldots, IMF_N$, where N is the number of IMFs. These IMFs are then soft-thresholded, yielding $tIMF_1, \ldots, tIMF_N$, which are thresholded versions of the original components. The filtered signal is obtained as a linear summation of thresholded IMFs.

A very common strategy used in the filtering procedure based on wavelets is to use the soft-thresholding technique described in [14]. The same idea is used for thresholding IMFs. For each IMF from 1 to N a threshold, $t_n, n = 1, \ldots, N$, is selected and soft-thresholding is applied to individual IMFs.

The threshold t_n is estimated by using the following strategy: a window of noise is selected from the original signal and then the boundaries of this window are used to extract regions of noise from IMFs. The standard deviation of each of those regions is then estimated, and

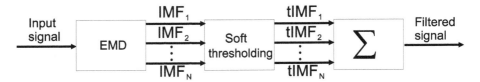

Figure 6. The EMD method is employed for decomposing the input signal into IMFs ($IMF_1, \ldots, IMF_N$, where N is the number of IMFs). These IMFs are soft-thresholded, yielding $tIMF_1, \ldots, tIMF_N$, which are thresholded versions of the original components. The filtered signal is obtained as a linear summation of thresholded IMFs.

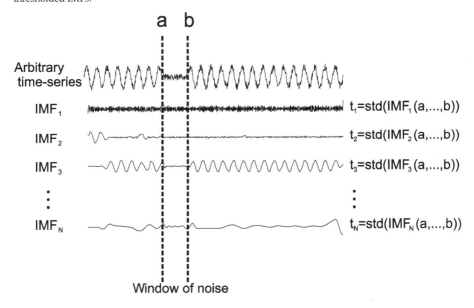

Figure 7. Illustrative example showing the estimate of thresholds t_n. First, a window of noise (i.e. samples within the interval [a,b]) is selected from the arbitrary time-series. The interval [a,b] is employed for selection of noise in the IMFs, and then from each IMF, thresholds $t_1, \ldots, t_N$ are defined. Note that *std* is the standard deviation.

these are regarded as the required thresholds ($t_1, \ldots, t_N$). Figure 7 illustrates the procedure for estimating t_n.

3.2.3. An example of application of the filter based on the EMD method

In this section, an example illustrating the application of the procedure for filtering EMG signals based on the EMD is provided. For this, the experimental surface electromyographic signal shown in Figure 8 is used.

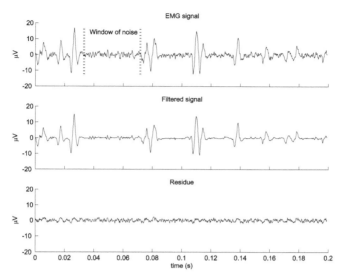

Figure 8. EMG signal and its filtered version. The residue, which is the difference between those signals is also shown.

The first step of the algorithm is to use the EMD (or sifting process) to decompose the experimental signal into intrinsic mode functions. Eight IMFs ($IMF1, \ldots, IMF8$) are obtained and they are presented in Figure 9(a).

The subsequent step is to threshold the components $IMF1, \ldots, IMF8$. Equation 4 was employed for denoising individual IMFs. The results of this procedure are shown in Figure 9(b). Note that in order to estimate thresholds for IMFs the boundaries of the window of noise (0.03 s and 0.07 s) indicated in Figure 8 were selected.

In the last step, the resulting (de-noised) components were combined to generate a filtered version of the original signal as shown in Figure 8. In the same figure, the residue, which is the difference between the original and filtered signals, is also presented. The random nature of this component and the attenuation of the noise in the EMG signal is apparent.

4. A system for extraction and visualization of MUAPs

The visual inspection of data is an important stage in signal analysis. It may help the investigator to identify relevant features, outliers and noise in the signal. Although visualization is an important and basic stage in data processing, in practice, its execution may be rather complex, specially when performed manually and the data lie in a high dimensional manifold.

In this context tools or systems that allow for an automatic visualization of signals play an important role. First, they significantly reduce the overall processing time of data, and

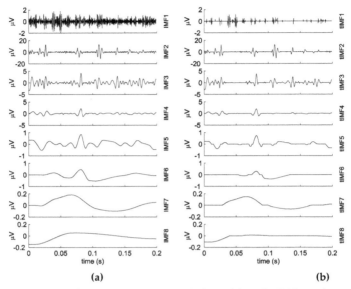

Figure 9. (a) Intrinsic mode functions ($IMF1, \ldots, IMF8$) obtained from the EMG signal presented in Figure 8. (b) De-noised intrinsic mode functions.

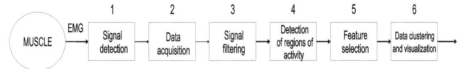

Figure 10. Block diagram of the system for extraction and visualization of MUAPs. After detection (1) and acquisition (2) the EMG signal is filtered (3), and signal windows, designated as regions of activity (RA), are extracted from it (4). In (5) features are selected from RA and then employed for their clustering and visualization.

secondly they may reveal information present in the signal which might be barely perceived in a manual analysis.

This section describes a system that can be used for the extraction and visualization of motor unit action potentials from electromyographic signals. It is formed by several basic units which are illustrated in Figure 10. Its input is a raw electromyographic signal, and its output is the visualization of MUAPs or any other information (e.g. noise) present in the signal grouped into logical units (clusters). This visualization allows the researcher to identify outliers, noise and groups of MUAPs. Each of the stages of this system is described below.

Once the EMG signal is detected it is amplified and digitized. An EMG amplifier[2] and data acquisition board[3] are important elements that contribute to the correct collection of data.

---

[2] Typical requirements of the signal conditioner are CMRR > 80 dB, input impedance > 10^{15} Ω, noise level < 1.2 μV.

[3] A possible model would be PC-card DAS 16/16 Measurement Computing

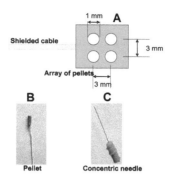

Figure 11. Types of electrodes for EMG signal detection. (A) A customized array of pellet electrodes. (B) Example of a single pellet electrode. (C) Concentric needle electrode.

Other relevant units include force sensors for monitoring the level of muscle contraction and biofeedback systems that provide a stimulus and information for subjects about the required task to be executed during the experiment.

4.1. System description

4.1.1. Signal detection and acquisition

The stage of signal detection will convert current generated by movement of ions (a physiological process) into current generated by movement of electrons (an electrical process). The choice of the type of electrode to be employed is dependent on the aim of the investigation. For instance, if the interest is to extract and visualize activity of motor unit action potentials from EMG signals, then needle electrodes are traditionally employed, mainly because of the high spatial resolution offered by these sensors. In fact, when studying the state of deep muscles this is the only possible choice. However, many studies [5, 11, 17, 43, 49] have shown that surface EMG electrodes with a sufficiently small contact surface may be successfully applied to the detection of MUAP activity in superficial muscles.

The system depicted in Figure 10 has been tested with two types of electrodes for signal detection. They are shown in Figure 11. One is a concentric needle electrode and the other is a customized array of pellet(surface) electrodes whose dimensions follow specifications provided in [43]. Both electrodes are passive and leads connecting them to the amplifier are shielded in order to attenuate the presence of spurious noise activity.

The use of pellet electrodes was a very cheap and simple solution for high spatial resolution signal detection, which yielded outstanding results and consistent detection of EMG signals.

4.1.2. Signal filtering

The main aim of this stage is to reduce the background activity present in electromyographic signals. This is relevant because high levels of background activity (noise) may affect the

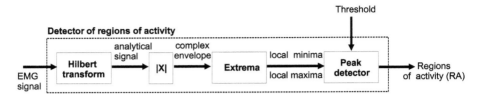

Figure 12. Block diagram of the detector of regions of activity.

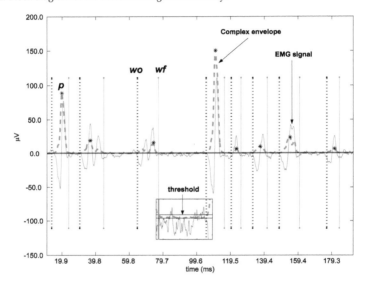

Figure 13. Example of detection of regions of activity. The experimental surface EMG signal and its complex envelope are shown. w_o and w_f are respectively the beginning and end of a region of activity. The peak (p) within each RA is marked with * and it is used as a reference point for feature selection. The inset shows a window of noise with the pre-defined threshold level.

detection of useful information (e.g. MUAPs). This stage may be performed by the filtering procedure based on the Empirical Mode Decomposition described above.

4.1.3. Detection of regions of activity

Following the stage of signal filtering the EMG signal is segmented into small windows, so-called regions of activity (RA), that may contain the activity of single MUAPs, MUAP overlaps or noise. A detector of RA was devised for extraction of RA from EMG signals. The block diagram of this is shown in Figure 12 and an example of its application is provided in Figure 13. Its input may be either a raw or filtered EMG signal and the output is a set of regions of activity.

Basically, this system will estimate the signal envelope and it will select from it reference points which define the beginnings and ends of RAs. Intuitively, the envelope is the overall shape of the amplitude of the signal and its use instead of the raw signal may simplify, in terms of practical implementation, the solution for this problem, mainly because the signal envelope is positive. For instance, a unique positive threshold may be employed for selection of RAs which are above it.

The envelope of time domain signals can be computed by low pass filtering and curve fitting techniques [21], or by using the Hilbert transform to compute the analytic signal [13]. The signal envelope generated from the first two methods is dependent on the choice of parameters like the filter order and the method for data fitting, whereas in the latter strategy no a priori parameters should be set before calculation of the signal envelope. For this reason this is the method implemented in this system, that is, the absolute value of the complex analytic signal (also known as the complex envelope [13]) is used to estimate the signal envelope.

From the signal envelope, local minima and local maxima points are estimated. This will reduce the number of candidate points to be searched by the peak detector. As a consequence, the processing time will also be reduced, which may be relevant for the analysis of either long or oversampled time-series. Another benefit of this stage is that noise activity may be eliminated.

The role of the peak detector is to search for extrema points which are above or below a threshold. Once a maximum (w_o) is found, the mean of the small window, $h_o = w_o + u$, is estimated and only if this mean is above the pre-defined threshold, w_o will be selected as the beginning of an RA. In this system u is set to 1 ms. Note that the analysis of the mean of h_o may avert the selection of spurious activity (e.g. noise). The end of an RA is detected when a minimum (w_f) is found. In this case, w_f is considered to be valid only if the mean of the window $h_o = w_o - u$ is below the threshold.

The threshold, th, is estimated as $th = k \times std(W_{noise})$, where W_{noise} is a window of noise directly selected from the analysed signal, $std(W_{noise})$ is the standard deviation of W_{noise}, and k is a user-defined constant which controls the threshold level. A typical value for k is 5. It is supported by the Chebyshev theorem [26]. This theorem states that, for any distribution, if $k > 1$ then the fraction of observations that fall within a range of $\pm k \times std(W_{noise})$ around the mean is at least $F = 1 - (1/k^2)$. For instance, $F = 0.96$ for $k = 5$, which means in practice that any sample within the interval $[mean(W_{noise}) - k \times std(W_{noise}), mean(W_{noise}) + k \times std(W_{noise})]$ has a 96% chance of really being noise.

4.1.4. Feature selection

In the feature selection stage, features will be selected for use in data clustering from a window within the region of activity. Figure 14 shows reference points in time (w_o, p_o, p, p_f, w_f) for definition of this window.

w_o and w_f are respectively the time when the region of activity starts and ends. These points are estimated by the detector of regions of activity. p is the time when the highest peak in the

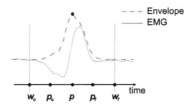

Figure 14. Identification of reference points in time for feature selection. w_o and w_f indicate the beginning and end of the region of activity. p is the time when the highest peak in the envelope and within the interval $[w_o, w_f]$ occurs, and p_o and p_f define the boundaries of a rectangular window for feature selection.

envelope of the RA occurs. This point is also the point where the variation in amplitude of the signal is maximal within the RA. This is illustrated in Figure 13.

p_o and p_f are respectively the beginning and end of the window to be selected for analysis. These points are defined as follows: $p_o = p - min\{t_o, p - w_o\}$ and $p_f = p + min\{t_o, w_f - p\}$, with t_o set to 2 ms. Note that the width of the window defined by p_o and p_f may vary for different RAs. Therefore, interpolation (splines) was employed for selection of 40 samples from each window defined in the interval $[p_o, p_f]$. This means that after feature selection each pattern is represented by a 40D vector with samples obtained via an interpolation procedure.

4.1.5. Data visualization and clustering

In order to ease the application of the sequence of steps detailed in Figure 10 a graphical user interface (GUI) was devised. The main GUI is shown in Figure 15. The system is capable of importing EMG data organized in columns of a text file and storing them in user-defined variables which are available in a list box. The main interface is organized into four logical sections (tabs) that should be accessed sequentially.

Figure 16 shows the module which allows the user to filter the EMG signal. The filtering procedure based on the Empirical Mode Decomposition is available here. The result of the automatic detection of regions activity is given in the interface shown in Figure 17.

The results of the data clustering and visualization step are presented in the GUI shown in Figure 18. At this stage patterns are clustered by means of Generative Topographic Mapping (GTM) and data visualization is performed with the GTM grid [3, 9]. For generation of the GTM grid, a GTM model with 25 Gaussian functions and 16 basis functions with a width of 1 is fitted to the data. The data can also be projected onto the two-dimensional space so that the user can visualize the distances of distinct groups of MUAPs (see Figure 19).

5. The application of EMG decomposition in the treatment of neuromuscular disorders triggered by stroke

Stroke, or cerebrovascular accident (CVA), affects a great number of individuals, and is the leading cause of disability among adults [10, 24]. After the event, most individuals must deal with severe reduction of motor functionality [31].

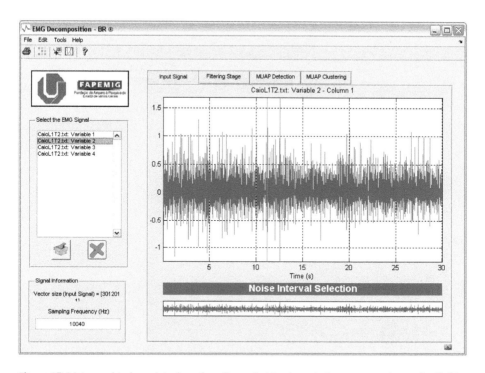

Figure 15. Main graphical user interface of a software that implements the sequence of steps detailed in Figure 10.

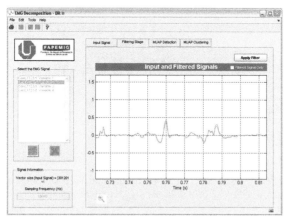

Figure 16. Graphical user interface which allows the user to filter the input signal.

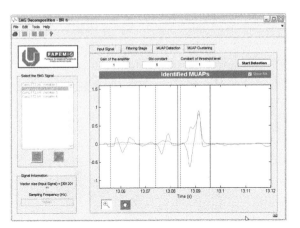

Figure 17. Automatic detection of regions of activity.

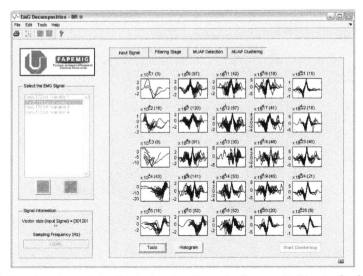

Figure 18. Data clustering and visualization based on Generative Topographic Mapping [3, 9].

Hemiplegia and spasticity are among the most common post-stroke motor deficits. In general, hemiplegia is characterized by an initial flaccid stage, with motor and sensory losses, in which the patient finds himself unable to sustain or move the affected limb. In many cases, the motor sequel evolves into spasticity, a stage characterized by muscle hypertonia. Hemiplegia and spasticity are closely related to the disuse of the affected limb and to secondary changes in muscles, such as: selective atrophy of fast twitch type II muscle fibers, abnormal recruitment

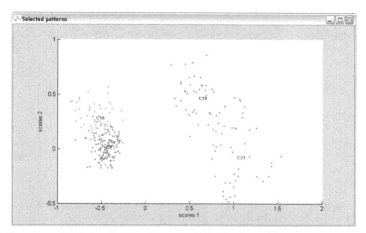

Figure 19. Two-dimensional visualization of groups of MUAPs obtained from the application of Principal Component Analysis.

of motor units, muscle contractures, and decreased cortical representation, due to disuse of the affected limb [28].

Several rehabilitation therapies have been used in an attempt to recover motor functionality, especially for upper limbs. The majority is based on the premise that the neural system can be retrained [20, 34]. The ability of the neural system to adapt to a new structural and functional condition, as well as its response to a traumatic destructive injury or to subtle changes resulting from the processes of learning and memory, is called 'neuroplasticity" [1, 12].

Recent studies have shown that behavioral experiments, important tools used in rehabilitation strategies based biofeedback techniques, have a strong impact on the motor cortical representation post-stroke. In this sense, we can also infer that it is possible to use biofeedback strategies for the modulation of neural plasticity, seeking the recovery of motor skills in rehabilitation protocols. The question is: how can we generate the appropriate information for feedback in a situation where the encephalic damage is manifested by an uncontrolled recruitment, or the lack of recruitment, of muscle fibers - leading to involuntary muscle hypotonia or hypertonia? Looking for a solution to this problem, a novel strategy, based in the assessment of the recruitment rate of motor units, is under test (see [39]), to generate control information for a multimodal biofeedback system. In this approach, instead of simply evaluating the process of muscle contraction, the researches decided to focus on the neural control over the muscles. However, the information regarding the recruitment of motor units are not readily available through standard surface EMG. Hence, the biofeedback relies heavily on a robust EMG decomposition system.

The strategy addressed by [39] is based on the discrimination and feature extraction of EMG signals (Motor Unit Action Potential) in order to control a virtual device. The biofeedback protocol immerses the patient in a virtual reality environment in which a representation of the affected limb will be presented. This virtual member is controlled according to the pattern of motor unit recruitment. Thus, although the spastic or hemiplegic patient lacks of proper voluntary control, it is expected that the system will be able to capture small voluntary changes in motor recruitment, as a result of his desire to do so. These changes can then be used to guide the movements of the virtual member. In so doing, the virtual feedback operates as a guide, indicating that the current mental strategy (neuromotor control) is correct and should be encouraged, reinforcing the process of neural reorganization (neuroplasticity).

6. Future directions

The widespread use of automatic tools for decomposing EMG signals is dependent on how easy is to detect MUAPs from the surface of the skin, on the identification of new applications, either online or offline, which might employ the results of the EMG decomposition, and also on the sharing and availability of developed tools to clinicians and researchers.

Ideally the sensors used for detecting MUAPs from the surface of the skin should be easy of applying and using. As a number of applications require the use of multiple sensors organized on an array the solution to this issue becomes more complex. Therefore, further research on this area, with the aim of developing sensors that allow for the reproduction of experiments is required.

Most applications found in the area of EMG decomposition are solely focused on the development of the automatic tool for decomposing the EMG signal, or in the classification and discrimination of MUAPs. Therefore, the identification of new useful applications are required in order to disseminate the relevance of the technique to other areas. For instance, the use of motor unit information could be employed in robotics, myofeedback, and human-machine interface development.

A major limitation of the results in the area of EMG decomposition is that the developed tools are not shared by researchers. The sharing of these tools together with EMG signal databases could be beneficial to the widespread use of the tools. Furthermore, this would allow researchers to objectively compare distinct solutions.

Considering the application of artefact removal from biomedical signals, the development of algorithms for reducing the influence of noise over signals in real time, without a priori knowledge about the origins and characteristics of the noise, are required. In this way the application of adaptive techniques such as Empirical Mode Decomposition should be further exploited.

It is also expected that the use of these filters can be part of the solution of the problem of EMG decomposition by directly decomposing the raw EMG signal into its motor unit action potential trains. If such filters are developed, EMG decomposition tools could be embedded in hardware speeding up the results from multichannel data.

Acknowledgements

The authors would like to express their gratitude to the Research Foundation of the State of Minas Gerais (FAPEMIG), The National Council for Scientific and Technological Development (CNPq) and the Coordination for the Improvement of Higher Education Personnel (CAPES).

Author details

Adriano O. Andrade and Alcimar B. Soares
Faculty of Electrical Engineering, Laboratory of Biomedical Engineering, Federal University of Uberlândia, Uberlândia, Brazil

Slawomir J. Nasuto
School of Systems Engineering, University of Reading, Reading, United Kingdom

Peter J. Kyberd
Institute of Biomedical Engineering, University of New Brunswick, Fredericton, Canada

7. References

[1] I Adams. Comparison of synaptic changes in the precentral and postcentral cerebral cortex of aging humans: a quantitative ultrastructural study. *Neurobiology of Aging*, 8:203–12, 1987.

[2] Metin Akay. *Biomedical signal processing*. Academic Press, Inc, San Diego, California, 1st edition, 1994.

[3] Adriano O Andrade. *Decomposition and Analysis of Electromyographic Signals*. PhD thesis, University of Reading, Reading, UK, 2005.

[4] Adriano O Andrade, Peter J Kyberd, and Slawomir J Nasuto. Time-frequency analysis of surface electromyographic signals via Hilbert spectrum. In Serge H Roy, Paolo Bonato, and Jens Meyer, editors, *XVth ISEK Congress - An Invitation to Innovation*, page 68.

[5] Adriano O Andrade, Peter J Kyberd, and Slawomir J Nasuto. The application of the Hilbert spectrum to the analysis of electromyographic signals. *Information Sciences*, 178(9):2176–2193, 2008.

[6] Adriano O Andrade, Peter J Kyberd, and Sean D Taffler. A novel spectral representation of electromyographic signals. In Ron S. Leder, editor, *Engineering in Medicine and Biology Society - 25th Annual International Conference*, volume 1, pages 2598–2601. IEEE.

[7] Adriano O Andrade, Slawomir J Nasuto, and Peter J Kyberd. EMG signal filtering based on empirical mode decomposition. *Biomedical Signal Processing and Control*, 1(1):44–55, 2006.

[8] Adriano O Andrade, Slawomir J Nasuto, and Peter J Kyberd. Extraction of motor unit action potentials from electromyographic signals through generative topographic mapping. *Journal of the Franklin Institute*, 344(3-4 (May-July)):154–179, 2007.

[9] Adriano O Andrade, Slawomir J Nasuto, Peter J Kyberd, and Catherine M Sweeney-Reed. Generative topographic mapping applied to clustering and visualization of motor unit action potentials. *Biosystems*, 82(3):273–84, 2005.

[10] American Heart Association. Heart disease and stroke statistics — 2011 update: a report from the american heart association. *Circulation*, 123:e18–e209, 2011.

[11] Alfredo Avellido and Adriano O Andrade. Determination of feature relevance for the grouping of motor unit action potentials through a generative mixture model. *Biomedical Signal Processing and Control*, 2:111–121, 2007.

[12] S N Burke and C A Barnes. Neural plasticity in the ageing brain. *Nature Reviews Neuroscience*, (7):30–40, 2006.

[13] Lokenath Debnath and Piotr Mikusinski. *Introduction to Hilbert Spaces with applications.* Academic Press, San Diego, CA, second edition, 1999.

[14] David L Donoho. De-noising by soft-thresholding. *IEEE Transactions on Information Theory,* 41(3):613–627, 1995.

[15] H Etawil and Daniel W Stashuk. Resolving superimposed motor unit action potentials. *Medical and Biological Engineering and Computing,* 34(1):33–40, 1996.

[16] Jianjun Fang, Gyan C Agarwal, and Bhagwan T Shahani. Decomposition of multiunit electromyographic signals. *IEEE Transactions on Biomedical Engineering,* 46(6):685–697, 1999.

[17] Gonzalo A. Garcia, Kenzo Akazawa, and Ryuhei Okuno. Decomposition of surface electrode-array electromyogram of biceps brachii muscle in voluntary isometric contraction. In *Engineering in Medicine and Biology Society - 25th Annual International Conference,* pages 2483–2486. IEEE.

[18] Tamara Grujic and Ana Kuzmanic. Denoising of surface emg signals: a comparison of wavelet and classical digital filtering procedures. *Technology and Healthcare,* 12(2):130–135, 2004.

[19] Mohamed H Hassoun, Chuanming Wang, and A Robert Spitzer. NNERVE: Neural network extraction of repetitive vectors for electromyography - part I: Algorithm. *IEEE Transactions on Biomedical Engineering,* 41(11):1039 – 1051, 1994.

[20] Koichi Hiraoka. Rehabilitation effort to improve upper extremity function in post-stroke patients: A meta-analysis. *Journal of Physical Therapy Science,* 13:5–9, 2001.

[21] Norden E Huang, Zheng Shen, Steven R Long, Manli C Wu, Hsing H Shih, Quanan Zheng, Nai-Chyuan Yen, Chi Chao Tung, and Henry H Liu. The empirical mode decomposition and the Hilbert spectrum for nonlinear and non-stationary time series analysis. *Proceedings of Royal Society of London,* 454:903–995, 1998.

[22] R S LeFever and Carlo J De Luca. A procedure for decomposing the myoelectric signal into its constituent action potentials–part I: Technique, theory, and implementation. *IEEE Transactions on Biomedical Engineering,* 29(3):149–57, 1982.

[23] M. Lei and G. Meng. Classification of the action surface emg signals based on the dirichlet process mixtures method. volume 7101 LNAI of *4th International Conference on Intelligent Robotics and Applications, ICIRA 2011,* pages 212–220. Aachen, 2011.

[24] I Lessa. Epidemiologia das doenças cerebrovasculares no brasil. *Revista da Sociedade de Cardiologia do Estado de Sao Paulo,* 4:509–518, 1999.

[25] Michael S Lewicki. A review of methods for spike sorting: the detection and classification of neural action potentials. *Comput. Neural Syst.,* 9:R53 – R78, 1998.

[26] H Lohninger. *Teach/Me Data Analysis.* Springer-Verlag, Berlin, Germany, 1999.

[27] Carlos J De Luca. Decomposition of the EMG signal into constituent motor unit action potentials. *Muscle Nerve,* 18(12):1492–4, 1995.

[28] L Lundy-Ekman. *Neurociencias: fundamentos para reabilitaçao,* pages 155–199. Elsevier, Rio de Janeiro, 2008.

[29] Bruno Mambrito and Carlo J. De Luca. A technique for the detection, decomposition and analysis of the EMG signal. *Electroencephalography and clinical neurophysiology,* 58:175–188, 198

[30] H. R. Marateb, S. Muceli, K. C. McGill, R. Merletti, and D. Farina. Robust decomposition of single-channel intramuscular emg signals at low force levels. *Journal of Neural Engineering*, 8(6), 2011.

[31] N E Mayo, S Wood-Dauphinee, S Ahmed, C Gordon, J Higgins, S McEwen, and N Salbach. Disablement following stroke. *Disabil. Rehabil.*, 21(5-6):258–268, 1999.

[32] Kevin C. McGill, Kenneth L. Cummins, and Leslie J. Dorfman. Automatic decomposition of the clinical electromyogram. *IEEE Transactions on Biomedical Engineering*, BME-32(7):470–477, 1985.

[33] Michel Misiti, Yves Misiti, Georges Oppenheim, and Jean-Michel Poggi. *Wavelet toolbox user's guide*. The Mathworks, Inc, third edition, 2004.

[34] Susan O'Sullivan and Thomas Schmitz. *Fisioterapia: Avaliaçao e Tratamento*. Manole, 2010.

[35] H. Parsaei and D. W. Stashuk. A method for detecting and editing mupts contaminated by false classification errors during EMG signal decomposition. 33rd Annual International Conference of the IEEE Engineering in Medicine and Biology Society, EMBS 2011, pages 4394–4397.

[36] H. Parsaei and D. W. Stashuk. SVM-based validation of motor unit potential trains extracted by EMG signal decomposition. *IEEE transactions on biomedical engineering*, 59(1):183–191, 2012.

[37] Constantinos S Pattichis and Marios S Pattichis. Time-scale analysis of motor unit action potentials. *IEEE Transactions on Biomedical Engineering*, 46(11):1320 – 1329, 1999.

[38] G. L. Sheean. Quantification of motor unit action potential energy. *Clinical Neurophysiology*, 123(3):621–625, 2012.

[39] M B Silva, D Viera, Ângela A R de Sá, and Alcimar Barbosa Soares. Proposta de treinamento com biofeedback eletromiográfico em ambiente de realidade virtual como apoio a reabilitaçao motora após acidente vascular encefálico. In *2o Congresso Brasileiro de Eletromiografia e Cinesiologia, COBEC 2012*, pages 1–3.

[40] Daniel W Stashuk. Decomposition and quantitative analysis of clinical electromyographic signals. *Med Eng Phys*, 21(6-7):389–404, 1999.

[41] Daniel W Stashuk and G M Paoli. Robust supervised classification of motor unit action potentials. *Medical and Biological Engineering and Computing*, 36:75–82, 1998.

[42] Daniel W Stashuk and Y Qu. Adaptive motor unit action potential clustering using shape and temporal information. *Medical and Biological Engineering and Computing*, 34(1):41–9, 1996.

[43] Tzyh-Yi Sun, Thy-Sheng Lin, and Jia-Jin Chen. Multielectrode surface EMG for noninvasive estimation of motor unit size. *Muscle and Nerve*, 22:1063 – 1070, 1999.

[44] S Usui and I Amidor. Digital low-pass differentiation for biological signal processing. *IEEE Transactions on Biomedical Engineering*, 29:686–693, 1982.

[45] N. W. Willigenburg, A. Daffertshofer, I. Kingma, and J. H. van Dieën. Removing ecg contamination from emg recordings: A comparison of ica-based and other filtering procedures. *Journal of electromyography and kinesiology*, 2012.

[46] Zhengquan Xu and Shaojun Xiao. Digital filter design for peak detection of surface EMG. *Journal of Electromyography and Kinesiology*, 10:275–281, 2000.

[47] F. Zaheer, S. H. Roy, and C. J. De Luca. Preferred sensor sites for surface emg signal decomposition. *Physiological Measurement*, 33(2):195–206, 2012.

[48] Daniel Zennaro, Peter Wellig, Volker M. Koch, George S. Moschytz, and Thomas Laubli. A software package for the decomposition of long-term multichannel EMG signals using wavelet coefficients. *IEEE Transactions on Biomedical Engineering*, 50(1):58–69, 2003.

[49] Ping Zhou, Zeynep Erim, and W Z Rymer. Motor unit action potential counts in surface electrode array EMG. In *Engineering in Medicine and Biology Society - 25th Annual International Conference*, pages 2067–2070. IEEE.

Chapter 4

Sphincter EMG for Diagnosing Multiple System Atrophy and Related Disorders

Ryuji Sakakibara, Tomoyuki Uchiyama, Tatsuya Yamamoto, Fuyuki Tateno, Tomonori Yamanishi, Masahiko Kishi and Yohei Tsuyusaki

Additional information is available at the end of the chapter

1. Introduction

One of the hallmarks in the pathology of multiple system atrophy (MSA) is neuronal loss in the sacral Onuf's nucleus[11,33,37]. Onuf's nucleus plays a key role in urinary and fecal continence[12]. Neurons in this nucleus receive not only cortical inputs, but also noradrenergic and serotonergic facilitatory inputs via interneurons from various brainstem structures, including the pontine urine-storage center[57,68]. External anal sphincter (EAS)-electromyography (EMG) is an established method to detect neurogenic change in motor unit potentials (MUP), which mostly reflects denervation and reinnervation of the sphincter muscle[30]. The significance of the EAS-EMG in MSA has been well known[30,69,74]. Physiologically, external urethral sphincter (EUS) and EAS share sacral pudendal innervation from Onuf's nucleus[20]. In this article, we review the normal physiology and pathophysiology of the lower urinary tract and the lower gastrointestinal tract briefly, the current methods and interpretations of EAS or EUS-EMG, and sphincter EMG in autonomic disorders.

2. Physiology and pathophysiology of the lower urinary tract

The lower urinary tract consists of two major components, the bladder and urethra. The bladder is abundant with muscarinic M2,3 receptors (contraction) and adrenergic beta 3 receptors (relaxation)[12]. The urethra is abundant with adrenergic alpha 1A/D receptors (contraction) and nicotinic receptors (contraction) **(Fig. 1)**. The storage and emptying functions need an intact neuraxis that involves almost all parts of the nervous system[48]. This is in contrast to postural hypotension, which arises due to lesions below the medullary circulation center[56].

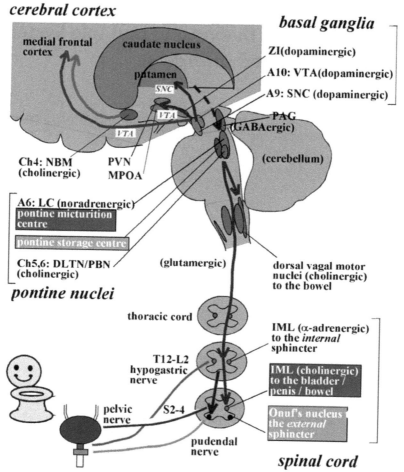

The lower urinary tract consists of two major components, the bladder and the urethra. The bladder is mainly innervated by the parasympathetic pelvic nerve. The urethra is innervated by the sympathetic hypogastric nerve and somatic pudendal nerve, respectively. Urinary storage is dependent on the reflex arc of the sacral spinal cord. The storage reflex is thought to be tonically facilitated by the brain, particularly the pontine storage center. The storage function is thought to be further facilitated by the hypothalamus, cerebellum, basal ganglia, and frontal cortex. Central cholinergic fibers from the nucleus basalis Meynert (NBM, also called the Ch4 cell group) seem to facilitate urinary storage. Micturition is dependent on the reflex arc of the brainstem and spinal cord, which involves the midbrain periaqueductal gray (PAG) and the pontine micturition center (located in or adjacent to the locus coeruleus [LC]). The voiding function is thought to be initiated by the hypothalamus and prefrontal cortex, which overlap the storage-facilitating area.

PVN: paraventricular nucleus, MPOA: medial preoptic area, A: adrenergic/noradrenergic, ZI: zona incerta, VTA: ventral tegmental area, SNC: substantia nigra pars compacta, DLTN: dorsolateral tegmental nucleus, PBN: parabrachial nucleus, IML: IML cell column, GABA: γ-aminobutyric acid, T: thoracic, L: lumbar, S: sacral (cited from ref. 41)

Figure 1. Neural circuitry relevant to micturition.

Urinary storage is dependent on the autonomic reflex arc of the sacral cord[12]. This reflex is tonically facilitated by the brain, particularly the pontine storage center,[7,57] hypothalamus, cerebellum, basal ganglia, and frontal cortex[25]. In contrast, micturition is dependent on the autonomic reflex arc of the brainstem and spinal cord[12]. This reflex involves the periaqueductal gray[12,32,78] and the pontine micturition center (PMC)[6,7,12,54,63]. The PMC facilitates the sacral bladder preganglionic nucleus by glutamate[35], while inhibiting the sacral Onuf's nucleus by γ-amino-butyric acid (GABA) and glycine[8]. This reflex is regulated by the hypothalamus and prefrontal cortex[16,25].

Bladder (detrusor) overactivity is the major cause of urinary urgency/frequency and urgency incontinence[66]. In lesions above the brainstem, detrusor overactivity is considered an exaggerated micturition reflex[66]. This is in line with the fact that detrusor overactivity appearing after experimental stroke requires mRNA synthesis in the PMC[83]. The exaggeration of the micturition reflex might be brought about not only by decreased inhibition of the brain (by central cholinergic and D1 dopaminergic mechanisms); that is, it might be further facilitated by glutamatergic and D2 dopaminergic mechanisms[82]. Underactive detrusor (or bladder weakness) is the major cause of voiding difficulty in autonomic disorders. Underactive detrusor results from lesions in either upper or lower neurons innervating the bladder muscles, but typically occurs from lower neuron lesions.[1,48]

Urinary urgency incontinence and voiding difficulty in MSA result mostly from detrusor overactivity and underactive detrusor, respectively.[1,48] Patients with MSA often have a combination of detrusor overactivity in the filling phase and underactive detrusor in the voiding phase; this is called detrusor hyperactivity with impaired contractile function (DHIC). DHIC presumably reflects multiple lesions in both the storage-facilitating areas (the basal ganglia, pontine storage center) and the voiding-facilitating areas (the PMC, sacral preganglionic neurons in the intermediolateral [IML] cell columns) of this disorder.[23,79] In MSA, incomplete emptying is thought to be secondary to IML involvement.

Sphincter dysfunction contributes to voiding difficulty and urinary incontinence in autonomic disorders, although less commonly than over- or underactive detrusor does. When the urethral sphincter does not relax properly during voiding bladder contraction, it is called detrusor-sphincter dyssynergia.[1] Since a coordinated micturition reflex (bladder contraction with sphincter relaxation) needs an intact brainstem–sacral cord axis,[12] disruption of the axis (such as lesions affecting the cervical/thoracic spinal cord) may lead to detrusor–sphincter dyssynergia. Sphincter weakness is a cause of urinary incontinence. Sphincter weakness occurs from lesions in the sacral motoneurons (Onuf's nucleus), and typically appears in women with MSA as severe stress incontinence[49] or continuous urinary incontinence[34].

3. Physiology and pathophysiology of the lower gastrointestinal tract

The enteric nervous system plays the most important role in regulating the peristaltic reflex of the lower gastrointestinal tract[20]. Two types of myoelectrical activity or pressure changes in the colon are documented. Slow phasic pressure waves are the most common manometric phenomenon[26], and in humans are measured as spontaneous phasic rectal contraction[9,22]. The peristaltic reflex can be evoked by surface stroking or by circumferential stretching.[20] The reflex consists of two components: ascending contraction (mediated by cholinergic fibers) oral to the stimulus site, and descending relaxation (mediated by non-adrenergic, non-cholinergic fibers) caudal to the stimulus site[2].

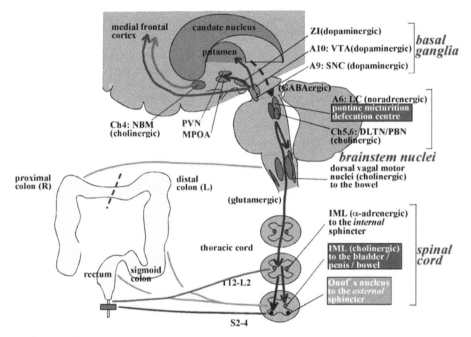

The function of the lower gastrointestinal tract is thought to depend on the brain and spinal cord, although less significantly than the lower urinary tract (LUT) does. Whereas the small intestine and ascending colon are innervated by the vagus nerves originating in the medulla, the descending colon, sigmoid colon, and rectum primarily share sacral innervation of the LUT (Figure 1). Both the sacral cord and the vagus nuclei receive projecting fibers from Barrington's nucleus (the pontine micturition/defecation center). Bowel function seems to be modulated by the higher brain structures, including the frontal lobe, the hypothalamus, and the basal ganglia; the main action of the latter on the bowel seems to be inhibitory.

NBM: nucleus basalis Meynert, Ch: cholinergic, PVN: paraventricular nucleus, MPOA: medial preoptic area, ZI: zona incerta, A: adrenergic/noradrenergic, VTA: ventral tegmental area, SNC: substantia nigra pars compacta, LC: locus ceruleus, DLTN: dorsolateral tegmental nucleus, PBN: parabrachial nucleus, PAG: periaqueductal gray, IML: IML cell column, GABA: γ-aminobutyric acid, T: thoracic, L: lumbar, S: sacral
(cited from ref. 41)

Figure 2. Neural circuitry relevant to defecation.

Other types of pressure changes in the colon include giant motor complexes[20]. A giant motor complex is a cyclic contractile activity with a periodicity of 20 to 30 min, and is perhaps analogous to the migrating motor complex of the small intestine[26]. A combination of slow waves and giant motor complexes is thought to promote bowel transport, which in humans is measured by colonic transit time[4]. The strength of cholinergic transmission in the enteric nervous system is thought to be regulated by opposing receptors; serotonin 5-HT4 receptor-mediating excitation[31,73] and dopamine D2 receptor-mediating inhibition[76].

Whereas the rostral lower gastrointestinal tract is innervated by the vagus nerves originating in the medulla, extra-enteric innervation of the caudal lower gastrointestinal tract primarily shares the innervation of the lower urinary tract **(Fig. 2)**[12,22]. The lower urinary tract and lower gastrointestinal tracts perform similar functions of storage and emptying. However, they differ profoundly with regard to anatomy (closed bag versus open-ended tube, respectively), luminal contents (liquid versus half-solid), and physiology (dysfunctional transport, rare ureter versus common bowel; smooth muscle contraction, bladder contraction only on emptying versus persistent spontaneous phasic rectal contraction; abdominal strain, minimal on urination versus strong on defecation)[22]. In addition, while the lower urinary tract requires an intact neuraxis for storage and emptying[12], it has not been entirely clear to what extent the lower gastrointestinal tract needs the extra-enteric nervous system.

Constipation in MSA most probably results from slow colonic transit, decreased phasic rectal contraction, and weak abdominal strain.[58] Some patients also have paradoxical sphincter contraction on defecation (PSCD).[58] The sites responsible for this dysfunction seem to be both the central and peripheral nervous systems, which regulate the lower gastrointestinal tract. Slow colonic transit and decreased phasic rectal contraction most probably reflect peripheral enteric nervous system lesions, whereas weak abdominal strain and PSCD may reflect central lesions.[61] In contrast, fecal incontinence results mostly from a weak anal sphincter due to denervation.[58]

4. Physiology and pathophysiology of the genital organ

The genital organ primarily shares lumbosacral innervation with the lower urinary tract. Erection is a vascular event[3]; occurring secondarily after dilatation of the cavernous helical artery and compression of the cavernous vein to the tunica albuginea[3]. Helical artery dilatation is brought about by activation of cholinergic and nitrergic nerves; this activation facilitates nitric oxide secretion from the vascular endothelium. Ejaculation is brought about by contraction of the vas deferens and the bladder neck, in order to prevent retrograde ejaculation, by activation of adrenergic nerves **(Fig. 3)**. Sacral Onuf's nucleus innervates the bulbocavernosus muscle; and is thought to participate in erection and ejaculation. Sexual intercourse in healthy men can be divided into 3 phases[65]: a) desire (libido), b) excitement and erection, and c) orgasm, seminal emission from the vas deferens, and ejaculation from the penis. Erection can be further classified into 3 types by the relevant stimulation: 1) psychogenic erection (by audiovisual stimulation), 2) reflexive erection (by somatosensory stimulation), and 3) nocturnal penile tumescence (NPT) (associated with rapid eye movement [REM]-sleep). 'Morning erection' is considered the last NPT in the nighttime.

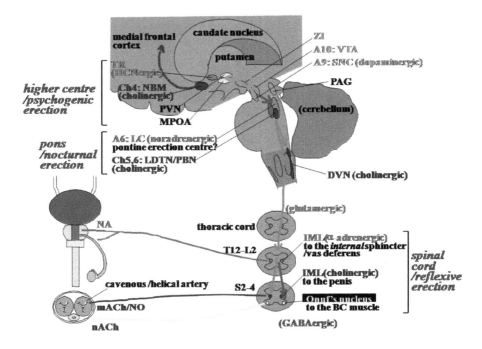

PAG, periaqueductal gray; LC, locus coeruleus; NBM, nucleus basalis Meynert; PVN, paraventricular nucleus; MPOA, medial preoptic area; A, adrenergic/noradrenergic; ZI, zona incerta; VTA, ventral tegmental area; SNC, substantia nigra pars compacta; DLTN, dorsolateral tegmental nucleus; PBN, parabrachial nucleus; IML, intermediolateral nucleus; GABA, γ-aminobutyric acid; T, thoracic; L, lumbar; S, sacral; NA, noradrenaline; Ach, acetylcholine; NO, nitric oxide. See text.

Figure 3. Neural circuitry relevant to erection.

Among the 3 types of erection, reflexive erection requires an intact sacral cord, particularly the intermediolateral (IML) cell columns. Pathology studies have shown that involvement of the IML nucleus is common in MSA, whereas it is uncommon in Parkinson's disease. Therefore, reflexive erection can be affected in patients with MSA. In patients with a supra-sacral spinal cord lesion, reflexive erection might be preserved, whereas psychogenic erection is severely disturbed because of a lesion in the spinal pathways to the sacral cord. Libido and erection are thought to be regulated by the hypothalamus; particularly the medial preoptic area (MPOA) and the paraventricular nucleus (PVN).[13,72] Recent neuroimaging studies have shown that penile stimulation or watching pornography activated these areas in humans[70]. NPT[15] seems to be regulated by the hypothalamic lateral preoptic area,[21] raphe nucleus, and locus ceruleus. Oxytocinergic neurons in the hypothalamic PVN are thought to facilitate erection by projecting directly to the sacral cord, and by projecting to the midbrain periaqueductal gray and the Barrington's nucleus (identical to the PMC).

In experimental animals, dopamine is known to facilitate erection and mating behaviors[13]. The MPOA/PVN receives projections from the nigral dopaminergic neurons. Prolactinergic neurons are thought to be inhibitory in sexual function. Prolactin-producing pituitary tumors often cause gynecomastia and erectile dysfunction in male patients. Hyperprolactinemia occurs after the use of sulpiride, metoclopramide, and chlorpromazine (all dopamine receptor antagonists). Therefore, dopaminergic neurons seem to facilitate oxytocinergic neurons whereas they inhibit prolactinergic neurons.

5. Methods and interpretations of sphincter EMG

In humans, the EUS and EAS share sacral pudendal innervation from Onuf's nucleus.[12,20] The EAS lies around the anal canal and forms an 8-shaped sphincter system on the pelvic floor **(Fig. 4)**. Although injury to the peripheral nerves may lead to the dysfunction of the EUS alone, lesions of the sacral Onuf's nucleus affect both the EAS and EUS. For this reason, we use EAS-EMG to assess urinary incontinence, as it is easier to perform and less painful than EUS-EMG. For the same reason, few studies have utilized EUS-EMG.[14,17] In women, the EUS muscle can be examined using a perineal approach. Examination of this muscle is more difficult in men; we can approach it with the fingers by feeling for the prostate within the rectum. However, EUS should be chosen in cases exhibiting a decelerating burst ('whale noise') with complex repetitive discharge in Fowler's syndrome.[24]

The EAS can be divided into a deep part (thick; around the rectal neck to the anal canal) and a subcutaneous part (thin; around the anus). The deep EAS is a major constituent in the generation of anal pressure to hold feces in when the rectum is full. The normal range of static anal pressure is more than 40 cmH$_2$O, and that of anal squeeze pressure is more than 50 cmH$_2$O.[22] The former is thought to reflect hypogastric adrenergic innervation, whereas the latter reflects somatic Onuf's nucleus innervation.[22] The subcutaneous EAS is easy to examine. It is reached by inserting a needle about 1 cm from the anal orifice, to a depth of 3–6 mm.[43]

Although the EAS is a skeletal muscle, it usually fires continuously during both waking and sleeping states. To assess EAS, an EMG computer with quantitative, template-operated MUP analysis software is recommended. The commonly used amplifier filter setting is 5–10 kHz. The tip of a concentric needle usually monitors an area approximately 500 micrometers in diameter, which includes approximately 20 MUPs. To assess acute denervation, insertion and spontaneous activities are checked as with the evaluation of other skeletal muscles. When the muscle is completely denervated, the EMG becomes silent. After an interval of 10–20 days, the insertion potentials become prolonged and abnormal spontaneous muscle activities, e.g., fibrillation potentials and positive sharp waves, appear. However, in the EAS, due to the continuous firing activities, it is not easy to see denervation potentials. In such cases, examination of the bulbocavernosus muscle has been recommended[44].

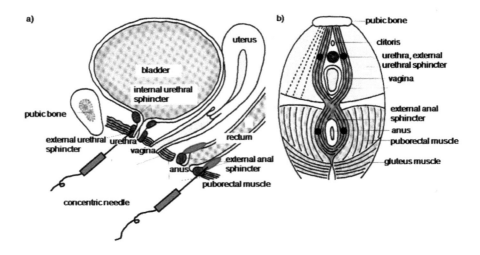

This figure illustrates where to insert concentric needles to measure external sphincter EMG.

Figure 4. The external anal sphincter and the external urethral sphincter.

A normal MUP usually has a 50–500 microV amplitude, a 3–8 msec duration, and 2–4 phases. In order to assess reinnervation, usually 10–20 single MUPs are recorded, which are automatically provided by an EMG computer. To ascertain single MUP, we still check each wave manually and adjust the onset and offset of each wave. It is particularly important to include late components (satellite potentials) to measure the duration of each unit.[42] When the muscle is chronically denervated, an intact nerve tends to innervate the adjacent denervated muscle fibers. As a result, MUPs become of high amplitude, of long duration, and polyphasic. Among various EMG parameters, the use of duration, MUP area, and number of turns is recommended for optimal diagnostic power (sensitivity and specificity) in the EAS muscle.[45] In addition, the results are dependent on the methods used; e.g., including or excluding late components. Palace et al. proposed that either of two criteria is sufficient to diagnose neurogenic changes in the EAS-EMG: (*a*) more than 20% of MUPs have a duration > 10 msec, or (*b*) the average duration of MUPs > 10 msec, particularly including the late components.[38] When satellite potentials were excluded, the duration of MUPs did not differ significantly between Parkinson's disease and MSA.[48] When lower motor neuron-type abnormalities are not apparent, it is reported that abnormal MUP recruitment pattern suggests pyramidal tract involvement.[18] In addition to MUP analysis in the external sphincter muscles, other neurophysiologic tests, e.g., pudendal nerve conduction, sacral reflexes, somatosensory evoked potentials and cranial magnetic stimulation, and urodynamic studies, can be of particular value in the study of autonomic patients.[29,40,41]

6. Sphincter EMG in autonomic disorders

6.1. MSA

Cardiovascular autonomic failure in MSA is thought to derive from neuron loss in the thoracolumbar intermediolateral (IML) cell columns of the spinal cord and the medullary circulation center. In contrast, lower urinary tract disorder in MSA is thought to reflect multiple lesions in the basal ganglia and the pontine storage center (storage-facilitating areas), as well as in the pontine micturition center in or adjacent to the locus ceruleus and the sacral IML cell columns (voiding-facilitating areas).[11] In addition, a distinguishing pathology in MSA is neuronal cell loss in the sacral Onuf nucleus.[33,37]

The first reports on neurogenic changes of EAS-EMG in MSA are attributed to Sakuta et al. (1978).[62] Since then, EAS-EMG results for over 500 MSA patients have been reported, with abnormality rates of more than 70% in many studies[5,30,36,38,47,53,62,64,71]. EAS-EMG is better tolerated and yields identical results to those from EUS investigation[5]. Abnormalities have also been recorded in the bulbocavernosus muscles in MSA.[67] In a larger study, Beck et al. (1994) reported that all (100%) 62 MSA patients with urological symptoms had abnormalities in both EAS and EUS-EMG.[5] Palace et al. (1997) reported abnormal EAS-EMG in 103 (82%) of 126 patients with MSA[38]. Chandiramani et al. (1997) found abnormal EAS-EMG in 49 (94%) of 52 patients with MSA[10]. Kirchhof et al. (1999) found abnormal EAS-EMG in 89 (91%) of 98 patients with MSA[28]. Sakakibara et al. (2000) found an abnormal EAS-EMG in 53 (74%) of 71 MSA patients[52]. These abnormalities correspond to selective loss of ventral horn cells and astrogliosis; the loss is particularly severe in the second and third sacral segments (Onuf's nucleus) in MSA[11]. Sphincter EMG has been proposed as a means of distinguishing between MSA and idiopathic Parkinson's disease (as described below), since the anterior horn cells of Onuf's nucleus are not affected in idiopathic Parkinson's disease.[10] In contrast, there have been debates about whether or not sphincter EMG can be used to distinguish MSA from idiopathic Parkinson's disease. In a study of 13 patients with idiopathic Parkinson's disease and 10 patients with MSA, Giladi et al. (2000) found significant overlap in all EMG parameters (presence of fibrillation potentials, MUP duration, presence of satellite potentials, percentage of polyphasic potentials)[19]. However, the durations of MUPs in both the MSA and Parkinson's disease groups were longer than in other studies.

It is reported that EAS-MUP abnormalities can distinguish MSA from idiopathic Parkinson's disease in the first 5 years after disease onset.[30,69,74] However, the prevalence of such abnormalities in the early stages of MSA has not been well known. In our recent study of 84 probable MSA cases, 62% exhibited neurogenic change.[80] The prevalence was relatively low presumably because up to 25% of our patients had a disease duration of 1 year or less. In such early cases, the diagnosis of MSA should be made with extreme caution. In addition to the clinical diagnostic criteria, we usually add an imaging study and we perform gene analysis to the extent possible. The prevalence of neurogenic change was 52% in the first year after disease onset, which increased to 83% by the fifth year (p<0.05) **(Fig. 5)**. Among the patients who underwent repeated studies, many had normal to mild abnormality at the initial examination, which turned into marked abnormality during the course of illness **(Fig. 6)**. Therefore, as expected, it is apparent that the involvement of Onuf's nucleus in MSA is time-dependent. In the early stages of illness, the prevalence of neurogenic change in MSA does not seem to be high. In 2 patients who underwent repeated studies, the EAS-EMG findings tended to remain normal. We do not know whether some MSA patients never develop neurogenic change during the course of their illness. However, Wenning et al. (1994) reported 3 patients with normal EAS-EMG and a postmortem confirmation of MSA.[77] Therefore, a negative result cannot exclude a diagnosis of MSA. More recently, Paviour et al. (2005) reported that among 30 sets of clinical data and postmortem confirmation in MSA cases with a duration of more than 5 years, 24 (80%) had abnormal EAS-EMG, 5 (17%) had a borderline result, and only 1 had a normal EMG.[39]

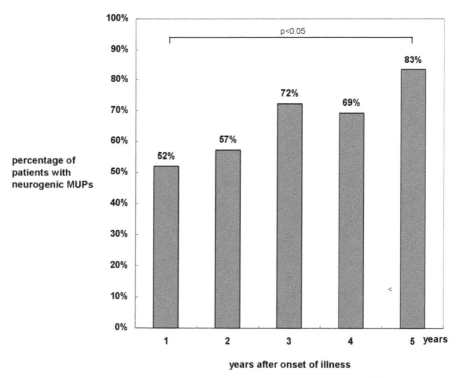

The prevalence of neurogenic sphincter EMG increased during the course of illness.
MUP: motor unit potential
(cited from ref. 74)

Figure 5. Neurogenic sphincter EMG and duration of illness.

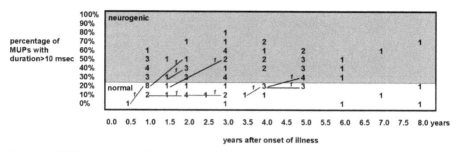

Percentage of MUPs with duration > 10 msec: one of two categories for neurogenic sphincter EMG.
straight figures: the number of patients
oblique figures: the number of patients who underwent the study repeatedly
MUP: motor unit potential
(cited from ref. 74)

Figure 6. Percentage of MUPs with duration > 10 msec and duration of illness.

The prevalence of neurogenic change also increased with the severity of gait disturbance ($p<0.05$) in our study. However, neurogenic change was not related to postural hypotension (reflecting adrenergic nerve dysfunction); erectile dysfunction in men (presumably reflecting cholinergic and nitrate oxidergic nerve dysfunction); detrusor overactivity (reflecting the central type of detrusor dysfunction); constipation (presumably reflecting both peripheral and central types of autonomic and somatic dysfunction); or gender (**Table 1**). The neurogenic change in EAS-MUP was slightly more common in those with detrusor-sphincter dyssynergia (reflecting the central type of sphincter dysfunction). It has been reported that neurogenic change does not correlate directly with a clinically obvious functional deficit.[74] Patients with marked abnormalities in EAS-MUP may have no faecal incontinence,[77] although, in such patients, anal sphincter weakness is not uncommon.[58] In our study, the prevalence of neurogenic change slightly increased with the severity of storage disorder (incontinence). The most common type of urinary incontinence in MSA is urgency incontinence, which results mostly from detrusor (bladder) overactivity. However, we noted urinary incontinence in 17 patients without detrusor overactivity or low-compliance detrusor; in those cases, the urinary incontinence may have had a sphincter etiology. Urinary incontinence was more severe in the patients with neurogenic change than in those without it ($p<0.05$).

We recently retrospectively analysed 445 case records of EMG cystometry with pressure flow studies, single motor unit potential (MUP) analysis in patients with parkinsonian syndrome, e.g., MSA: n=267, Parkinson's disease (PD): n=129, Dementia with Lewy bodies (DLB): n=25, and progressive supranuclear palsy (PSP): n=24. We carried out receiver operating characteristics (ROC) analysis, revealing that an area under the ROC curve (AUC) in differentiating MSA from other parkinsonian syndrome was 0.70 in duration, 0.62 in phase and 0.51 in amplitude, respectively, with statistically significance. Therefore, duration of MUPs is most sensitive for the differentiation of MSA among MUPs parameters.

	Patients with neurogenic sphincter EMG			Patients with neurogenic sphincter EMG		
	No	%		No	%	
Male	27/42	65	Female	25/42	59	NS
Age <60 years	22/39	56	Age >60 years	30/45	66	NS
MSA-C	29/50	58	MSA-P	23/34	68	NS
Independent walking (1-3*)	11/23	48	Wheelchair bound(6-7*)	9/11	82	p<0.05
Postural hypotension −	30/48	63	Postural hypotension +	22/36	60	NS
Constipation −	40/66	61	Constipation +	12/18	67	NS
Erectile dysfunction −	4/5	80	Erectile dysfunction +	19/30	63	NS
Continent	15/25	59	Incontinent	37/59	63	NS
RU <200 ml	36/62	58	RU >200 ml	16/22	73	NS
Detrusor overactivity −	14/26	55	Detrusor overactivity +	38/58	65	NS
UD/AD −	29/52	56	UD/AD +	20/32	63	NS
DSD −	44/73	60	DSD +	8/11	73	NS

*International cooperative ataxia rating scale, walking capacities subscale.
AD, acontractile detrusor; DSD, detrusor sphincter dyssynergy; MSA, multiple system atrophy; RU, residual urine volume; UD, underactive detrusor.

MSA: multiple system atrophy, RU: residual urine volume, UD: underactive detrusor, AD: acontractile detrusor
DSD: detrusor-sphincter dyssynergia
*: International Cooperative Ataxia Rating Scale, walking capacities subscale
(cited from ref. 74)

Table 1. Neurogenic sphincter EMG and clinical variables other than duration of illness.

6.2. Lewy body diseases

6.2.1. Idiopathic Parkinson's disease (IPD)

Several reports of "supposed IPD" have shown severe bladder dysfunctions, e.g., large post-void residuals or neurogenic change in the EAS-EMG. However, some of these reports were published before a definition of MSA was established. Recent studies have reported almost normal EAS-EMG in patients with typical IPD[38,47,53,67]. Stocchi's study (1997) is important, since EMG in patients with IPD and MSA was performed by researchers blinded to the diagnosis.[67] Pathological studies of IPD have shown a degenerative lesion in the spinal parasympathetic PGN[75], although the lesions are much less developed than those in MSA. No Lewy bodies were found in Onuf's nucleus innervating the anal sphincter in IPD.[75] In contrast, Libelius and Johansson (2000) described neurogenic change in EAS-EMG in PD after a disease duration of more than 5 years.[30] This remains a matter of controversy; on the other hand, some patients with DLB may show abnormal EAS-EMG, as described below.

6.2.2. Dementia with Lewy bodies (DLB)

DLB is characterized as dementia with fluctuating cognition and visual hallucination, with (sometimes atypical) parkinsonism. Cardiovascular and urinary autonomic failure is another feature. We performed urodynamic studies in 7 patients with DLB, and performed EAS-EMG in 3. Two of those 3 patients exhibited neurogenic changes in MUPs.[55]

6.2.3. Autonomic failure with Parkinson's disease (AFPD)

AFPD is an intermediate entity that describes a combination of autonomic failure and IPD, but without dementia. We performed urodynamic studies in 7 patients with AFPD and performed EAS-EMG in 4. Three of those 4 patients exhibited neurogenic changes in MUPs[55].

6.2.4. Pure autonomic failure (PAF)

Earlier studies reported normal EAS-EMG in small groups of patients with PAF. However, Ravits et al. (1996)[46] found abnormal EAS-EMG in 2 of 7 patients with PAF, although both of them were multiparous women. Sakakibara et al. performed urodynamic studies in 6 patients with PAF and EAS-EMG in 4. Three of those 4 patients exhibited neurogenic changes in MUPs.[51] In PAF, parkinsonism may appear after a 10-year interval.[81] Therefore PAF can be listed in the differential diagnosis of degenerative parkinsonism. To sum up, in all three Lewy body diseases (DLB, AFPD, PAF), the frequency of neurogenic changes seemed higher in EAS-EMG than in IPD but lower than in MSA. This suggests the involvement of the sacral Onuf's nucleus or its fibers in the external sphincter in these diseases. The prevalence of neurogenic changes in EAS-EMG seems to be: **MSA >> DLB = AFPD = PAF >> PD (Table 2)**. However, these assumptions require confirmation with a larger study. The results seem to be in accordance with the fact that 29% of the DLB patients undergoing EMG-cystometry had a low-compliance detrusor, indicating a pre-ganglionic lesion of the pelvic nerves. The bethanechol test showed that both of these patients had denervation supersensitivity of the detrusor, indicating a post-ganglionic lesion of the pelvic nerves. The results of physiological studies and metaiodobenzylguanidine (MIBG) cardiac scintigraphy suggested post-ganglionic abnormalities in DLB.

Disease	LUT symptoms	Urinary incontinence (storage dysfunction)	PVR> 100 ml (voiding dysfunction)	No. of patients	Reference	Detrus or overactivity (central type)	Low compliance (preGGL type)	Bethanechol supersensitivity (denervation) (postGGL type)	Neurogenic change of sphincter MUPs (denervation) (Onuf's nucleus)	No. of patients	Reference
MSA	96%	63%	52%	121	9	56%	31%	19%	93%	121	9, 11
DLB	100%	91%	27%	11	-	71%	29%	2/2	2/3	7	-
AFPD	100%	43%	29%	7	19	86%	14%	1/3	4/4	7	19
PAF	100%	33%	33%	6	17	67%	33%	2/3	¼	6	17
PD	53-70%	26-28%	0%	115	18	81%	0%	Not performed	5%	21	11

AFPD, autonomic failure with Parkinson's disease; DLB, dementia of Lewy body type; GGL, ganglion; LUT, lower urinary tract; MSA, multiple system atrophy; MUP, motor unit potential; PAF, pure autonomic failure; PD, Parkinson's disease; PVR, post-void residual.

MSA: multiple system atrophy, DLB: Dementia with Lewy bodies, AFPD: Autonomic failure with Parkinson's disease
PAF: Pure autonomic failure, PD: Parkinson's disease, GGL: ganglionic
(cited from ref. 78)

Table 2. Comparison of lower urinary tract function in DLB, AFPD, PAF, PD and MSA. See text.

6.3. Other parkinsonian disorders

6.3.1. Progressive supranuclear palsy (PSP)

We performed urodynamic studies in 9 patients with PSP and performed EAS-EMG in 4. Two of these 4 patients exhibited neurogenic changes in MUPs.[50] Abnormal sphincter EMG was also reported in 5 of 12 patients by Valldeoriola et al. (1995)[71], and in 2 of 8 patients by Palace et al. (1997)[38]. Libelius and Johansson (2000) also described anal sphincter EMG abnormalities in 2 of 3 patients with PSP.[30]

6.3.2. Corticobasal degeneration (CBD)

We performed urodynamic studies in 6 patients with CBD and EAS-EMG in 5 of them. However, none of the 5 patients showed neurogenic changes in the MUPs.[60] There is a considerable overlap in the clinical presentation of the parkinsonian form of MSA (MSA-P) and that of PSP. Therefore, we should be cautious in interpreting sphincter EMG in these disorders.

6.4. Cerebellar ataxia

6.4.1. Spinocerebellar ataxia 3 (SCA3)/Machado-Joseph disease

We performed urodynamic studies in 11 patients with spinocerebellar ataxia 3 (SCA3) and performed EAS-EMG in 9. Six of the 9 patients showed neurogenic changes in MUPs.[59]

6.4.2. Late cortical cerebellar atrophy (LCCA):

We performed urodynamic studies in 7 patients with LCCA, which is a pure cerebellar ataxia without heredity, and EAS-EMG in 3 of them. However, none of the 3 patients exhibited neurogenic changes in the MUPs.

6.4.3. Spinocerebellar ataxia 6 (SCA6)

We performed urodynamic studies in 9 patients with spinocerebellar ataxia 6 (SCA6) and performed EAS-EMG in 8. Five of the 8 patients showed neurogenic changes in MUPs.

6.5. Other diseases

Sakuta et al. performed EAS-EMG in 30 patients with amyotrophic lateral sclerosis (ALS).[62] None of them exhibited neurogenic changes in the MUPs, which contrasted with common neurogenic changes in the limb muscles in this disorder. These EMG findings correspond to the postmortem selective sparing of sacral Onuf's nucleus, which contrasts with severe loss of anterior horn cells innervating the limbs, tongue, and bulbar muscles[2]. Neurons in Onuf's nucleus demonstrate some morphological differences from the anterior horn cells innervating limb muscle [33]. However, more recent studies have shown abnormalities in the

Onuf's nucleus in most advanced cases with ALS[27], particularly in patients under mechanical ventilation.

7. Conclusions

We have reviewed the normal physiology and pathophysiology of the lower urinary tract and the lower gastrointestinal tract, the current methods and interpretations of sphincter EMG, and the application of this technique to various autonomic disorders. Sphincter EMG makes it easier to distinguish MSA from idiopathic Parkinson's disease in the first 5 years after disease onset, reflecting the significant involvement of the sacral spinal cord in MSA. However, abnormal sphincter EMG is also seen in some, though not many, patients with DLB or PSP. It is noteworthy that sphincter denervation leads to severe urinary and fecal incontinence in some female patients with MSA, which severely affects their quality of life. Sphincter EMG and relevant sacral autonomic tests are good diagnostic tools in autonomic disorders.

Author details

Ryuji Sakakibara*, Fuyuki Tateno, Masahiko Kishi and Yohei Tsuyusaki
Neurology, Internal Medicine, Sakura Medical Center, Toho University, Sakura, Japan

Tomoyuki Uchiyama and Tatsuya Yamamoto
Neurology, Chiba University, Chiba, Japan

Tomonori Yamanishi
Urology, Dokkyo Medical College, Tochigi, Japan

8. References

[1] Abrams P, Cardozo L, Fall M, Griffiths D, Rosier P, Ulmsten U, van Kerrebrock P, Victor A, Wein A (2002) The standardization of terminology of lower urinary tract function: report from the standardization sub-committee of the international continence society. Neurourol Urodynam 21: 167-178
[2] Amborova P, Hubkal P, Ulkova I, Hulin I (2003) The pacemaker activity of interstitial cells of cajal and gastric electrical activity. Physiol Res 52: 275-284
[3] Argiolas A, Melis MR (2005). Central control of penile erection: role of the paraventricular nucleus of the hypothalamus. Prog Neurobiol 76: 1-21.
[4] Bassotti G, Maggio D, Battaglia E, Giulietti O, Spinozzi F, Reboldi G, Serra AM, Emanuelli G, Chiarioni G (2000) Manometric investigation of anorectal function in early and late stage Parkinson's disease. J Neurol Neurosurg Psychiatry 68; 768-770
[5] Beck RO, Betts CD, Fowler CJ (1994) Genitourinary dysfunction in multiple system atrophy: clinical features and treatment in 62 cases. J Urol 151: 1336-1341.

---

* Corresponding Author

[6] Betts CD, Kapoor R, Fowler CJ (1992) Pontine pathology and voiding dysfunction. Br J Urol. 70: 100-102

[7] Blok BF, Holstege G (1999) The central control of micturition and continence: implications for urology. Br J Urol Int 83 Suppl 2: 1-6

[8] Blok BF, de Weerd H, Holstege G (1997) The pontine micturition center projects to sacral cord GABA immunoreactive neurons in the cat. Neurosci Lett 233: 109-112

[9] Broens P, Vanbeckevoort D, Bellon E, Penninckx F (2002) Combined radiographic and manometric study of rectal filling sensation. Dis Colon Rectum 45: 1016-1022

[10] Chandiramani VA, Palace J, Fowler CJ (1997) How to recognize patients with parkinsonism who should not have urological surgery. Br J Urol 80: 100 –104.

[11] Daniel SE (1992) The neuropathology and neurochemistry of multiple system atrophy. In Autonomic Failure, 3rd ed., R Bannister and CJ Mathias, eds. Oxford Medical Publications, Oxford, UK, 564-585

[12] de Groat WC (2006) Integrative control of the lower urinary tract: preclinical perspective. BJP 147: S25-S40

[13] Dominguez JM, Hull EM (2005). Dopamine, the medial preoptic area, and male sexual behavior. Physiol Behavior 86: 356-368.

[14] Eardley I, Quinn NP, Fowler CJ, Kirby RS, Parkhouse HF, Marsden CD, Bannister R. (1989) The value of urethral sphincter electromyography in the differential diagnosis of parkinsonism. Br J Urol 64: 360 –362

[15] Fisher C, Gross J, Zuch AJ (1965). Cycle of penile erection synchronous with dreaming (REM) sleep. Arch Gen Psychiatry; 12: 29-45.

[16] Fowler CJ (2006) Integrated control of lower urinary tract: clinical perspective. BJP 147: S14-S24

[17] Fowler CJ, Kirby RS, Harrison MJ, Milroy EJ, Turner-Warwick R. (1984) Individual motor unit analysis in the diagnosis of disorders of urethral sphincter innervation. J Neurol Neurosurg Psychiatry 47: 637-641

[18] Gilad R, Giladi N, Korczyn AD, Gurevich T, Sadeh M (2001). Quantitative anal sphincter EMG in multisystem atrophy and 100 controls. J Neurol Neurosurg Psychiatry. 71: 596-599.

[19] Giladi N, Simon ES, Korczyn AD, Groozman GB, Orlov Y, Shabtai H, Drory VE (2000) Anal sphincter EMG does not distinguish between multiple system atrophy and Parkinson's disease. Muscle Nerve 23: 731–734.

[20] Hansen MB (2003) Neurohumoral control of GI motility. Physiol Res 52: 1-30

[21] Hirschkowitz M, Schmidt MH (2005). Sleep-related erections: clinical perspectives and neural mechanisms. Sleep Med Rev 9: 311-329.

[22] Ito T, Sakakibara R, Uchiyama T, Liu Z, Yamamoto T, Hattori T (2006b) Videomanometry of the pelvic organs; a comparison of the normal lower urinary and GI tracts. Int J Urol 13: 29-35

[23] Ito T., Sakakibara R, Yasuda K, Yamamoto T, Uchiyama T, Liu Z, Yamanishi T, Awa Y, Yamamoto K, Hattori T (2006) Incomplete emptying and urinary retention in multiple system atrophy: when does it occur and how do we manage it? Mov Disord 21: 816-823

[24] Kavia RB, Datta SN, Dasgupta R, Elneil S, Fowler CJ. (2006) Urinary retention in women: its causes and management. BJU Int 97: 281-287
[25] Kavia RBC, Dasgupta R, Fowler CJ (2005) Functional imaging and the central control of the bladder. J Comp Neurol 493: 27-32
[26] Kellow JE, Delvaux M, Azpiroz F, Camilleri M, Quigley EMM, Thompson DG (1999) Principles of applied neurogastroenterology: physiology/motility-sensation. Gut 45; 17-24
[27] Kihira T, Yoshida S, Yoshimasu F, Wakayama I, Yase Y. (1997) Involvement of Onuf's nucleus in amyotrophic lateral sclerosis. J Neurol Sci 147: 81-88.
[28] Kirchhof K, Mathias CJ, Fowler CJ (1999) The relationship of uro-genital dysfunction to other features of autonomic failure in MSA. Clin Auton Res 9: 1–28.
[29] Lefaucheur JP (2006). Neurophysiological testing in anorectal disorders. Muscle Nerve. 33: 324-333.
[30] Libelius R, Johansson F (2000) Quantitative electromyography of the external anal sphincter in Parkinson's disease and multiple system atrophy. Muscle Nerve 23: 1250-1256
[31] Liu MT, Rayport S, Jiang L, Murphy DL, Gershon MD (2002) Expression and function of 5-HT3 receptors in the enteric neurons of mice lacking the serotonin transporter. Am J Physiol Gastrointest Liver Physiol 283: G1398-G1411
[32] Liu Z, Sakakibara R, Nakazawa K, Uchiyama T, Yamamoto T, Ito T, Hattori T (2004) Micturition-related neuronal firing in the periaqueductal gray area in cats. Neuroscience 126: 1075-1082
[33] Mannen T, Iwata M, Toyokura Y, Nagashima K (1982) The Onuf's nucleus and the external anal sphincter muscles in amyotrophic lateral sclerosis and Shy-Drager syndrome. Acta Neuropathol 58: 255-260
[34] Mashidori T, Yamanishi T, Yoshida K, Sakakibara R, Sakurai K, Hirata K. Continuous urinary incontinence presenting as the initial symptoms demonstrating acontractile detrusor and intrinsic sphincter deficiency in multiple system atrophy. Int J Urol. 14: 10; 972-974 2007
[35] Matsumoto G, Hisamitsu T, De Groat WC (1995) Role of glutamate and NMDA receptors in the descending limb of the spinobulbospinal micturition reflex pathway of the rat. Neurosci Lett 183: 58-61
[36] Nahm F, Freeman R (2003) Sphincter electromyography and multiple system atrophy. Muscle Nerve 28: 18-26.
[37] Onufrowicz B (1899) Notes on the arrangement and function of the cell groups in the sacral region of the spinal cord. J Nerv Ment Dis 26: 498-504
[38] Palace J, Chandiramani VA, Fowler CJ. (1997) Value of sphincter electromyography in the diagnosis of multiple system atrophy. Muscle Nerve 20: 1396-1403
[39] Paviour DC, Williams DC, Fowler CJ, Quinn NP, Lees AJ (2005) Is sphincter electromyography a helpful investigation in the diagnosis of multiple system atrophy? A retrospective study with pathological diagnosis. Mov Disord 20: 1425–1430.

[40] Pellegrinetti A, Moscato G, Siciliano G, Bonuccelli U, Orlandi G, Maritato P, Sartucci F (2003). Electrophysiological evaluation of genito-sphincteric dysfunction in multiple system atrophy. Int J Neurosci. 113: 1353-1369.

[41] Podnar S (2007). Neurophysiology of the neurogenic lower urinary tract disorders. Clin Neurophysiol. 118: 1423-1437.

[42] Podnar S, Fowler CJ. (2004) Sphincter electromyography in diagnosis of multiple system atrophy: technical issues. Muscle Nerve 29: 151–156

[43] Podnar S, Rodi Z, Lukanovic A, Trsinar B, Vodusek DB. (1999) Standardization of anal sphincter EMG: technique of needle examination. Muscle Nerve 22: 400-403

[44] Podnar S, Vodusek DB. (2001) Protocol for clinical neurophysiologic examination of the pelvic floor. Neurourol Urodyn 20: 669-682

[45] Podnar S. (2007) Neurophysiology of the neurogenic lower urinary tract disorders. Clin Neurophysiol. 118: 1423-1437

[46] Ravits J, Hallett M, Nilsson J, Polinsky R, Dambrosia J (1996). Electrophysiological tests of autonomic function in patients with idiopathic autonomic failure syndromes. Muscle Nerve. 19: 758-763.

[47] Rodi Z, Denislic M, Vodusek D (1996) External anal sphincter electromyography in the differential diagnosis of parkinsonism. J Neurol Neurosurg Psychiatry 60: 460-461.

[48] Sakakibara R, Fowler CJ (2001) Brain disease (Chapter 9). In: Seminars in Clinical Neurology (by World Federation of Neurology). Neurologic bladder, bowel, and sexual function. Edited by Fowler CJ, Elsevier, Boston, 229-243

[49] Sakakibara R, Hattori T, Kita K, Arai K, Yamanishi T, Yasuda K ： Stress-induced urinary incontinence in patients with spinocerebellar degeneration J Neurol Neurosurg Psychiatry 64: 3; 389-391 1998

[50] Sakakibara R, Hattori T, Tojo M, Yamanishi T, Yasuda K, Hirayama K (1993). Micturitional disturbance in progressive supranuclear palsy. J Auton Nerv Syst. 45: 101-106.

[51] Sakakibara R, Hattori T, Uchiyama T, Asahina M, Yamanishi T (2000). Micturitional disturbance in pure autonomic failure. Neurology. 54: 499-501.

[52] Sakakibara R, Hattori T, Uchiyama T, Kita K, Asahina M, Suzuki A, Yamanishi T (2000) Urinary dysfunction and orthostatic hypotension in multiple system atrophy: which is the more common and earlier manifestation? Neurol Neurosurg Psychiatry 68: 65–69.

[53] Sakakibara R, Hattori T, Uchiyama T, Yamanishi T (2001) Videourodynamic and sphincter motor unit potential analyses in Parkinson's disease and multiple system atrophy. J Neurol Neurosurg Psychiatry 71: 600-606.

[54] Sakakibara R, Hattori T, Yasuda K, Yamanishi T (1996) Micturitional disturbance and pontine tegmental lesion; urodynamic and MRI analyses of the vascular cases. J Neurol Sci 141: 105-110

[55] Sakakibara R, Ito T, Uchiyama T, Asahina M, Liu Z, Yamamoto T, Yamanaka Y, Hattori T (2005) Lower urinary tract function in dementia of Lewy body type (DLB). J Neurol Neurosurg Psychiatry 76: 729-732.

[56] Sakakibara R, Mori M, Fukutake T, Kita K (1997) Orthostatic hypotension in a case with multiple sclerosis. Clin Auton Res 7: 163-165

[57] Sakakibara R, Nakazawa K, Shiba K, Nakajima Y, Uchiyama T, Yoshiyama M, Yamanishi T, Hattori T (2002) Firing patterns of micturition-related neurons in the pontine storage centre in cats. Auton Neurosci Basic Clin 99: 24-30

[58] Sakakibara R, Odaka T, Uchiyama T, Asahina M, Yamaguchi K, Yamaguchi T, Yamanishi T, Hattori T (2004) Colonic transit time, sphincter EMG and rectoanal videomanometry in multiple system atrophy. Mov Disord 19: 924-929

[59] Sakakibara R, Uchiyama T, Arai K, Yamanishi T, Hattori T (2004). Lower urinary tract dysfunction in Machado-Joseph disease: a study of 11 clinical-urodynamic observations. J Neurol Sci. 218: 67-72.

[60] Sakakibara R, Uchiyama T, Yamanishi T, Hattori T (2004). Urinary function in patients with corticobasal degeneration; comparison with normal subjects. Neurourol Urodyn. 23: 154-158.

[61] Sakakibara R, Uchiyama T, Yamanishi T, Shirai K, Hattori T. (2008) Bladder and bowel dysfunction in Parkinson's disease. J Neural Transm 115: 443-460

[62] Sakuta M, Nakanishi T, Toyokura Y (1978) Anal muscle electromyograms differ in amyotrophic lateral sclerosis and Shy-Drager syndrome. Neurology 28: 1289-1293.

[63] Sasaki M (2005) Role of Barrington's nucleus in micturition. J Comp Neurol 493: 21-26

[64] Schwarz J, Kornhuber M, Bischoff C, Straube A. (1997) Electromyography of the external anal sphincter in patients with Parkinson's disease and multiple system atrophy: frequency of abnormal spontaneous activity and polyphasic motor unit potentials. Muscle Nerve 20: 1167–1172.

[65] Singer C, Weiner WJ, Sanchez-Ramos JR, Ackerman M (1989). Sexual dysfunction in men with Parkinson's disease. J Neurol Rehab 3: 199-204.

[66] Steers WD (2002) Pathophysiology of overactive and urge urinary incontinence. Rev Urol 4 Suppl 4: S7-S18

[67] Stocchi F, Carbone A, Inghilteri M, Monge A, Ruggieri S, Berardelli A, Manfredi M (1997) Urodynamic and neurophysiological evaluation in Parkinson's disease and multiple system atrophy. J Neurol Neurosurg Psychiatry 62: 507–511.

[68] Thor KB (2003) Serotonin and norepinephrine involvement in efferent pathways to the urethral rhabdosphincter: implications for treating stress urinary incontinence. Urology 62: 3-9

[69] Tison F, Arne P, Sourgen C, Chrysostome V, Yeklef F (2000) The value of external anal sphincter electromyography for the diagnosis of multiple system atrophy. Mov Disord 15: 1148-1157

[70] Tsujimura A, Miyagawa Y, Fujita K, Matsuoka Y, Takahashi T, Takao T, Matsumiya K, Osaki Y, Takasawa M, Oku N, Hatazawa J, Shigeo Kaneko S, Okuyama A (2006). Brain processing of audiovisual sexual stimuli inducing penile erection: a positron emission tomography study. J Urol 176: 679-683.

[71] Valldeoriola F, Valls-Sole J, Tolosa E, Marti M (1995) Striated anal sphincter denervation in patients with progressive supranuclear palsy. Mov Disord 10: 550–555.

[72] van Furth WR, Wolterink G, van Ree JM (1995). Regulation of masculine sexual behavior; involvement of brain opioids and dopamine. Brain Research Reviews 21: 162-184.

[73] 74   Vaughan CJ, Aherne AM, Lane E, Power O, Carey RM, O'Connell DP (2000) Identification and regional distribution of the dopamine D1A receptor in the GI tract. Am J Physiol Regulatory Integrative Comp Physiol 279: R599–R609

[74] Vodusek DB (2001)   Sphincter EMG and differential diagnosis of multiple system atrophy. Mov Disord 16: 600-607

[75] Wakabayashi K, Takahashi H (1997) Neuropathology of autonomic nervous system in Parkinson's disease. Eur Neurol. 38 Suppl 2: 2-7.

[76] Walker JK, Gainetdinov RR, Mangel AW, Caron MG, Shetzline MA (2000) Mice lacking the dopamine transporter display altered regulation of distal colonic motility. Am J Physiol Gastrointest Liver Physiol. 279: G311-318

[77] Wenning GK, Ben-Schlomo Y, Magalhaes M, Daniel S, Quinn N (1994) Clinical features and natural history of multiple system atrophy. Brain 117: 835-845.

[78] Yaguchi H, Soma H, Miyazaki Y, Tashiro J, Yabe I, Kikuchi S, Sasaki H, Kakizaki H, Moriwaka F, Tashiro K (2004)   A case of acute urinary retention caused by periaqueductal grey lesion. J Neurol Neurosurg Psychiatry 75; 1202-1203

[79] Yamamoto T, Sakakibara R, Uchiyama T, Liu Z, Ito T, Awa Y, Yamanishi T, Hattori T (2006)   Neurological diseases that cause detrusor hyperactivity with impaired contractile function. Neurourol Urodynam 25: 356-360

[80] Yamamoto T, Sakakibara R, Uchiyama T, Liu Z, Ito T, Awa Y, Yamanishi T, Hattori T (2005)   When is Onuf's nucleus involved in multiple system atrophy? A sphincter electromyography study. J Neurol Neurosurg Psychiatry 76: 1645-1648.

[81] Yamanaka Y, Asahina M, Hiraga A, Sakakibara R, Oka H, Hattori T. (2007) Over 10 years of isolated autonomic failure preceding dementia and Parkinsonism in 2 patients with Lewy body disease. Mov Disord 22: 595-597.

[82] Yokoyama O, Yoshiyama M, Namiki M, de Groat WC (2002) Changes in dopaminergic and glutamatergic excitatory mechanisms of micturition reflex after middle cerebral artery occlusion in conscious rats. Exp Neurol 173, 129-135

[83] Yokoyama O, Yotsuyanagi S, Akino H, Moriyama H, Matsuta Y, Namiki M (2003) RNA synthesis in pons necessary for maintenance of bladder overactivity after cerebral infarction in rat. J Urol. 169: 1878-1884

Chapter 5

The Usefulness of Mean and Median Frequencies in Electromyography Analysis

Angkoon Phinyomark, Sirinee Thongpanja, Huosheng Hu,
Pornchai Phukpattaranont and Chusak Limsakul

Additional information is available at the end of the chapter

1. Introduction

Rich useful information can be obtained from the muscles and researchers can use such information in a wide class of clinical and engineering applications by measuring surface electromyography (EMG) signals (Merletti & Parker, 2004). Normally, EMG signals are acquired by surface electrodes that are placed on the skin superimposed on the targeted muscle. In order to use the EMG signal as a diagnosis signal or a control signal, a feature is often extracted before performing analysis or classification stage (Phinyomark et al., 2012a) because a lot of information, both useful information and noise (Phinyomark et al., 2012b), is contained in the raw EMG data. An EMG feature is a distinct characteristic of the signal that can be described or observed quantitatively, such as being large or small, spiky or smooth, and fast or slow. Generally, EMG features can be computed in numerical form from a finite length time interval and can change as a function of time, i.e. a voltage or a frequency. They can be computed in several domains, such as time domain, frequency domain, time-frequency and time-scale representations (Boostani & Moradi, 2003). However, frequency-domain features show the better performance than other-domain features in case of the assessing muscle fatigue (Al-Mulla et al., 2012). Mean frequency (MNF) and median frequency (MDF) are the most useful and popular frequency-domain features (Phinyomark et al., 2009) and frequently used for the assessment of muscle fatigue in surface EMG signals (Cifrek et al., 2009).

This chapter presents a usefulness of MNF and MDF in electromyography analysis. The successful muscular fatigue assessment based on MNF and MDF methods is presented together with the principle and theory of MNF and MDF in this chapter, and also up-to-date literature reviews of MNF and MDF in the analysis of EMG signals. In order to analyse the EMG signals during dynamic movements, the effects of muscle force and muscle geometry (joint angle) should have paid more attention (Cechetto et al., 2001; Doheny et al., 2008). In the literature, such effects on MNF and MDF have still been inconclusive (Doheny et al., 2008; Phinyomark et al., 2012c). A summary of the conflicting results mentioned in the literature is also presented. The possible reasons for the conflicting results in both effects are discussed. In addition to the clinical applications, the classification of EMG signals during upper-limb movements for using in the engineering applications (Oskoei & Hu, 2007) is proposed in this chapter.

The rest of this chapter is as follows: Section 2 presents the principle and theory of MNF and MDF, and the relations between MNF (and MDF) and other EMG frequency-domain features are also described and discussed. In Section 3, the extensive review and careful survey of the up-to-date experiments for the assessing muscle fatigue using MNF and MDF in numerous applications are summarized, and moreover, the recent trend of MNF and MDF in the assessment of muscle fatigue is discussed in this section. On the other hand, the effects of muscle force and muscle geometry are described respectively in Section 4 and Section 5, with the re-evaluating results for both effects using the new EMG data set. In addition, a number of techniques that are possible to make the consistent results for both effects are suggested. In Section 6, the usefulness of MNF and MDF in the EMG pattern classification is proposed with the related works. The modified MNF and MDF in order to improve the robustness property for the classifying EMG signals are also presented. Lastly, the conclusion and future trends of using MNF and MDF to analyse EMG signals are presented in Section 7.

2. Principle and theory of mean and median frequencies

Frequency-domain or spectral-domain features are usually used in the assessing muscle fatigue and analysing MU recruitment (Oskoei & Hu, 2008). To transform the EMG signal in the time-domain to the frequency-domain, a Fourier transform of the autocorrelation function of the EMG signal is employed to provide the power spectrum (PS) or the power spectral density (PSD). Although PSD can be estimated by different methods, i.e. modern, parametric or model-based, the most commonly used PSD estimator in the EMG signal analysis is the Periodogram. It is defined as the square of absolute value of the Fourier transform of EMG signal divided by the signal length. Another stable and accurate PSD estimator is the autoregressive (AR) model (Zhang et al., 2010). Different kinds of statistical variables are applied to the PSD of EMG signal and the two popular used variables of PSD are mean and median. However, there are several possible statistical variables that can be applied to the PSD of EMG signal, such as summation or total, and peak value. Definitions of other statistical variables are presented in Section 2.2.

2.1. The definition of mean and median frequencies

MNF is an average frequency which is calculated as the sum of product of the EMG power spectrum and the frequency divided by the total sum of the power spectrum (e.g. Oskoei & Hu, 2008; Phinyomark et al., 2012a). MNF has a similar definition as several features, i.e.

the central frequency (f_c), centroid and the spectral center of gravity, in a number of studies (Du & Vuskovic, 2004; Farina & Merletti, 2000). In addition, MNF is also called as mean power frequency and mean spectral frequency in several works. The definition of MNF is given by

$$MNF = \sum_{j=1}^{M} f_j P_j \left/ \sum_{j=1}^{M} P_j \right. ,$$ (1)

where f_j is the frequency value of EMG power spectrum at the frequency bin j, P_j is the EMG power spectrum at the frequency bin j, and M is the length of frequency bin. In the analysis of EMG signal, M is usually defined as the next power of 2 from the length of EMG data in time-domain.

MDF is a frequency at which the EMG power spectrum is divided into two regions with equal amplitude (e.g. Oskoei & Hu, 2008; Phinyomark et al., 2012a). MDF is also defined as a half of the total power, or TTP (dividing the total power area into two equal parts). The definition of MDF is given by

$$\sum_{j=1}^{MDF} P_j = \sum_{j=MDF}^{M} P_j = \frac{1}{2} \sum_{j=1}^{M} P_j .$$ (2)

The behaviour of MNF and MDF is always similar. However, the performance of MNF in each of the applications is quite different compared to the performance of MDF, although both features are two kinds of averages in statistics. More details about the performance of both features are discussed in Section 3 to Section 6.

It should be noted that MNF is always slightly higher than MDF because of the skewed shape of EMG power spectrum (Knaflitz et al., 1990), whereas the variance of MNF is typically lower than that of MDF. In theory, the standard deviation of MDF is higher than that of MNF by a factor 1.253 (Balestra et al., 1988). However, the estimation of MDF is less affected by random noise, particularly in the case of noise located in the high frequency band of EMG power spectrum, and more affected by muscle fatigue (Stulen & De Luca, 1981).

2.2. The relations between mean and median frequencies and other EMG frequency-domain features

Other spectral variables that have been applied in the analysis of EMG signal are total power (TTP), mean power (MNP), peak frequency (PKF), the spectral moments (SM), frequency ratio (FR), power spectrum ratio (PSR), and variance of central frequency (VCF) (Phinyomark et al., 2012a). The definition of all variables is presented in the following.

1. TTP is an aggregate of EMG power spectrum (Phinyomark et al., 2012a). This feature is also defined as the energy and the zero spectral moment (SM0) (Du & Vuskovic, 2004). Its equation can be expressed as

$$TTP = \sum_{j=1}^{M} P_j = SM0 .$$ (3)

2. MNP is an average power of EMG power spectrum (Phinyomark et al., 2012a). It can be defined as

$$MNP = \sum_{j=1}^{M} P_j \Big/ M .$$ (4)

3. PKF is a frequency at which the maximum EMG power occurs (Phinyomark et al., 2012a). It can be expressed as

$$PKF = \max(P_j), \quad j=1, ..., M .$$ (5)

4. SM is an alternative statistical analysis way to extract feature from the power spectrum of EMG signal. Normally, the first three moments (SM1-SM3) are employed as the EMG features (Du & Vuskovic, 2004). Their equations can be defined as

$$SM1 = \sum_{j=1}^{M} P_j f_j; \ SM2 = \sum_{j=1}^{M} P_j f_j^2; \ SM3 = \sum_{j=1}^{M} P_j f_j^3 .$$ (6)

5. FR is used to discriminate between relaxation and contraction of the muscle using a ratio between low- and high-frequency components of EMG signal (Han et al., 2000; Phinyomark et al., 2012a). The equation is defined as

$$FR = \sum_{j=LLC}^{ULC} P_j \Big/ \sum_{j=LHC}^{UHC} P_j ,$$ (7)

where ULC and LLC are respectively the upper- and the lower-cutoff frequency of low-frequency band, and UHC and LHC are respectively the upper- and the lower-cutoff frequency of high-frequency band. The cutoff frequency between low- and high-frequencies can be defined by two ways: the experiment (Han et al., 2000) and the MNF value (Oskoei & Hu, 2006).

6. PSR is a ratio between the energy P_0 which is nearby the maximum value of EMG power spectrum and the energy P which is the whole energy of EMG power spectrum (Qingju & Zhizeng, 2006). It can be seen as an extended version of PKF and FR. The equation can be expressed as

$$PSR = \frac{P_0}{P} = \sum_{j=f_0-n}^{f_0+n} P_j \Big/ \sum_{j=-\infty}^{\infty} P_j ,$$ (8)

where f_0 is defined as the value of PKF and n is the integral limit.

7. VCF is defined by using a number of the spectral moments (SM0-SM2) and MNF. It can be computed by the following equation

$$VCF = \frac{1}{SM0}\sum_{j=1}^{M} P_j \left(f_j - MNF\right)^2 = \frac{SM2}{SM0} - \left(\frac{SM1}{SM0}\right)^2. \tag{9}$$

TTP, MNP, and SM are frequency-domain features that extract the same information as time-domain features based on the energy information (Phinyomark et al., 2012a). Hence, the discriminant of TTP, MNP and SM in space has the similar pattern as the time-domain features based on the energy information, i.e. integrated EMG (IEMG), root mean square (RMS), mean absolute value (MAV), and variance of EMG (VAR). Due to the fact that muscle fatigue results in an increase of EMG signal amplitude, time-domain features based on energy information, i.e. IEMG, MAV and RMS, can track this behaviour. Thus, TTP, MNP and SM can also be used as an indicator of muscle fatigue, although EMG signal amplitude, itself, is rarely used to detect muscle fatigue. However, these features can be used in a combination with the spectral analysis i.e. MNF and MDF. On the other hand, all spectral features except PSR have the different discriminant patterns in feature space compared with MNF and MDF. In case of $n = 20$, the pattern of PSR is an inverse case of MNF and MDF patterns (Phinyomark et al., 2012a).

3. Assessing the muscle fatigue using mean and median frequencies

Muscle fatigue is generally defined as an activity induced loss of the ability to produce force with the muscle. Usually, the muscle fatigue is a result of prolonged or repetitive works (De Luca, 1984). It should be noted that the usual term "muscle fatigue" is generally meaning in fact "local muscle fatigue" (Chaffin, 1973). Undetected fatigue for a long-time can cause injury to the subject and is often irreversible. If an automated muscle fatigue detection system in wearable technology was feasible, it could be employed as an indicator to reduce the chances of work-place injury and aid sporting performance (Al-Mulla et al., 2012). Among a number of sources and techniques (Al-Mulla et al., 2011), e.g. acoustic-myography (AMG), mechano-myography (MMG), near-infrared spectroscopy (NIRS), sono-myography (SMG) and ultrasound, the EMG signal is used even more often and has several advantages, such as a non-invasiveness, an ability to monitor fatigue of a particular muscle and a real-time muscle fatigue monitoring during the performance of defined work (Petrofsky et al., 1982).

The assessment of muscle fatigue with surface EMG signals can be applied in a wide class of applications, such as muscle fatigue during repeated cycling sprints (Hautier et al., 2000), muscle fatigue in children with cerebral palsy (Leunkeu et al., 2010), muscle fatigue during playing the PC games (Oskoei et al., 2008), and the low back pain in helicopter pilots (Balasubramanian et al., 2011). Several classical and modern signal processing techniques have been applied (Cifrek et al., 2009), such as the RMS, the zero-crossing rate (ZCR), the averaged instantaneous frequency, wavelet analysis, fractal analysis, and also MNF and MDF.

Among such techniques, MNF and MDF so far have been hailed as the gold standard for muscle fatigue assessment with surface EMG signals due to the fact that muscle fatigue results in a downward shift of frequency spectrum of the EMG signal. Moreover, during the fatigue of muscle, several changes have been found, i.e. a relative decrease in signal power at high-frequency, a small increase in signal power at low-frequency, an increase in spectrum slope at high-frequency, and a decrease in spectrum slope at low-frequency (Petrofsky et al., 1982; Sato, 1982; Viitasalo & Komi, 1977). There are several possible reasons for the changes in the EMG signal, such as the modulation of recruitment firing rate, the grouping and slowing of CV, and synchronization of the signal (De Luca, 1979; Hermens et al., 1984; Viitasalo & Komi, 1977).

Using MNF and MDF to detect muscle fatigue in static contractions is clearly known because during static contraction the EMG signals may be assumed to be stationary during short-time intervals (0.5-2s). On the other hand, in dynamic contractions, the EMG signal information has been changed as a function of time that cannot be analyzed by simply applying FFT and most recently EMG studies have been applied to the study of dynamic contraction. The instantaneous mean and median frequency (IMNF and IMDF) are introduced to fulfill the requirement (Roy et al., 1998) by using time-frequency or time-scale approaches, such as short-time Fourier transform (STFT) (Cifrek et al., 2000; Thongpanja et al., 2010, 2011), Wigner distribution (WD), Choi-Williams distribution (CWD) (Knaflitz & Bonato, 1999), time-varying autoregressive approach (TVAR) (Zhang et al., 2010), and continuous wavelet transform (CWT) (Karlsson et al., 2000).

Further, there are several ways to use IMNF and IMDF to detect muscle fatigue. For example, Georgakis et al. (2003) demonstrated that the performance of the average of IMNF and IMDF is better than the traditional MNF and MDF. On the other hand, a slope of the regression line that fits the maximum values of IMNF and IMDF during cyclic contractions is used as a fatigue index in Cifrek et al. (2000).

Many research works reported on the effectiveness of MNF and MDF applied to EMG signal as a mean of identifying muscle fatigue. The experimental conditions for several studies (based on literature published between 1980-2011) are summarized in Table 1. Most of the studies have been performed MNF and MDF to detect the muscle fatigue in primarily static muscle contraction but also in dynamic muscle contraction.

In Table 1, most of the studies recorded EMG data from 10 subjects and the volunteers between 20 and 30 years of age (young subjects) are the main target. However, in Masuda et al. (1999), age of the subjects is ranged from 19 to 73 years (both young and older subjects). EMG signals obtained from young and older subjects are quite different, as mentioned in Tavakolan et al. (2011) that the difference in classification accuracy obtained from the young and older subjects is approximately 7%. Although Kalra et al. (2012) found that MDF of EMG is not significantly impacted by age at 50-100%MVC of the BB muscle, the effect of age needs to be carefully considered in future research. In addition to the effect of age, the effect of gender is another factor that should be paid more an interest (Kalra et al., 2012).

Reference	N	Age	Muscle	ID	Force levels	RT	Filter
Petrofsky & Lind (1980b)	10	23.2±2.3	BR	40	25, 40, 70%MVC	F	-
Gerdle et al. (1990)	9	30-40	BB	-	20, 40, 60, 80, 100%MVC	-	-
Merletti & Roy (1996)	6	-	TA	-	50, 60, 70, 80%MVC	90-170	-
Mannion & Dolan (1996)	10	-	RF, VL	-	20, 30, 40, 50, 60%MVC	F	-
Potvin (1997)	15	24±3	BB	30	7kg	F	15-450
Masuda et al. (1999)	19	19-73	VL	5	50%MVC	F	5-1000
Rainoldi et al. (1999)	10	30.2±6.1	BB	10	10, 30, 50, 70%MVC	30	10-450
Cifrek et al. (2000)	10	22.9±1.5	RF, VL, VM	30	50%MVC	F	20-480
Bonato et al. (2001)	-	-	FDI	5	10%MVC	150	8-450
MacIsaac et al. (2001)	7	26±7	BB	40	20-30%MVC	F	1-1000
Arnall et al. (2002)	10	-	PS	-	40, 50, 60%MVC	60	-
Allison & Fujiwara (2002)	10	29.4±4.8	BB	25	60%MVC	C1	20-500
Bilodeau et al. (2003)	14	22-43	RF, VL, VM	20	100%MVC	C2	15-4000
Georgakis et al. (2003)	30	-	RF, VL, VM	20	60%MVC	60	10-500
Clancy et al. (2005)	12	31.4±11.1	FDS, ECR	-	10, 20, 30, 40, 50, 60, 70, 80, 90%MVC	F	25-1350
Ravier et al. (2005)	10	24±1.5	BB	75	70%MVC	F	2-600
Zaman et al. (2011)	11	24±4	BB	5	40%MVC	F	-
Soares et al. (2011)	10	24±2.8	BB	5	40%MVC	90	-

Table 1. A survey of the experimental conditions in related works about muscle fatigue assessment with surface EMG signals using MNF and MDF in chronological order. Note that N is the number of subjects; ID is the inter-electrode distance (mm); RT is the recording time (s); Filter is the specification of filtering (Hz); MVC is maximum voluntary contraction; F is the EMG data is recorded until the subject cannot support the required force level; C1 is the EMG data is recorded until force is below 35%MVC; C2 is the EMG data is recorded until force is below 50%MVC; BR is brachioradialis; BB is biceps brachii; TA is tibialis anterior; RF is rectus femoris; VL is vastus lateralis; VM is vastus medialis; FDI is first dorsal interossrous; PS is paraspinal; FDS is flexor digitorum superficialis; ECR is extensor carpi radialis.

The next interested factor in Table 1 is the recording time. Because in the analysis of muscle fatigue, the EMG signals recorded during the fatigue of muscle are needed. Most of the studies used a level of force as the threshold to finish the recording. In other words, the EMG data have been recorded until the subject cannot maintain the required force level. However, several studies define the specific recording times that range from 30s to 170s.

Other factors are varied, such as the inter-electrode distance (5-75 mm), the levels of force (10-100%MVC), and the specification of filtering (1-1350 Hz). However, most of the studies paid more an interest to the study of biceps brachii muscle. The evaluating performance between each pair of the methods and the muscles should be done in future study.

4. Effect of muscle force on mean and median frequencies

In order to make a reliably automate the muscle fatigue determination, the knowledge of the effects of time-varying factors on MNF and MDF is very important. Two time-varying factors, muscle force and muscle geometry, are the major factors due to the activities that involve dynamic muscle contractions (muscle force and/or geometry are changing) (Cechetto et al., 2001). It should be noted that the number and firing rate of active motor units (MUs) do not significantly affect MNF and MDF in both experimental and theoretical studies (Englehart & Parker, 1994; Solomonow et al., 1990).

The individual effects of muscle force and muscle geometry on MNF and MDF have been investigated in many previous researches. The effect of muscle force is discussed in this section, while the effect of muscle geometry will be discussed in the next section.

At present, the conflicting results of MNF and MDF with the muscle force effect exist in the literature. The difference in the experimental conditions for most of the studies is presented in Table 2. Maybe it is the possible reasons for the conflicting results of MNF and MDF on muscle force effect. It can be observed from the table that three different cases exist for the effect of muscle force on MNF and MDF.

- In the first case (CF1), MNF and MDF are unaffected or only weakly affected by changes in muscle force or load levels (Bilodeau et al., 1991; Cechetto et al., 2001; Hagberg & Ericsson, 1982; Inbar et al., 1986; Merletti et al., 1984; Petrofsky & Lind, 1980a, 1980b; Viitasalo & Komi, 1978).
- In the second case (CF2), MNF and MDF increase as muscle force levels increase (Doheny et al., 2008; Gander & Hudgins, 1985; Gerdle et al., 1990; Hagberg & Ericsson, 1982; Hagberg & Hagberg, 1989; Moritani & Muro, 1987; Muro et al., 1982; Van Boxtel & Schomaker, 1984).
- In the third case (CF3), MNF and MDF decrease as muscle force levels increase (Kaplanis et al., 2009; Rainoldi et al., 1999).

Each of the first two cases is found in eight publications, while the third case exists only in two publications. However, the third case is found in the most recent study (Kaplanis et al., 2009) which used the EMG data recorded from 94 subjects (the largest EMG data compared with other publications).

Reference	N	Age	Muscle	ID	Force levels	RT	Filter	CF
Viitasalo & Komi (1978)	7	-	RF,VL,VM	-	-	-	-	1
Petrofsky & Lind (1980a)	8	22-52	FCR	40	5-100%MVC	3	-	1
Petrofsky & Lind (1980b)	10	23.2±2.3	BR	40	10, 20, 40, 60, 80, 100%MVC	3	-	1
Hagberg & Ericsson (1982)	4	21-24	BB,BR,BL	20	5, 10, 15, 20, 25, 30, 40, 50, 80%MVC	3-5	0.2-2000	1,2
Muro et al. (1982)	5	32.5±8.2	BB	-	0.25, 0.5, 1, 2, 3kg	10	-	2
Merletti et al. (1984)	26	22.6±6.4	FDI	10	20, 80%MVC	3-5	30-350	1
Van Boxtel & Schomaker (1984)	19	18-32	FL,CS	15	20, 40, 60, 80%MA	3	3-520	2
Gander & Hudgins (1985)	6	20-40	BB	-	1-10Nm	8.2	-	2
Inbar et al. (1986)	9	30-40	BB,ED	35	30, 50, 70, 90%MVC	6	1-1000	1
Moritani & Muro (1987)	12	26.3±2.5	BB	6	0-80%MVC	5	<520	2
Hagberg & Hagberg (1989)	14	36±8	TZ	30	0-100%MVC	10-15	5-500	2
Gerdle et al. (1990)	9	30-40	BB	-	20, 40, 60, 80, 100%MVC	1-2	-	2
Bilodeau et al. (1991)	14	30.2±7.8	TB,AN	6	10, 20, 40, 60, 80%MVC	3	16-800	1
Rainoldi et al. (1999)	10	30.2±6.1	BB	10	10, 30, 50, 70%MVC	30	10-450	3
Cechetto et al. (2001)	12	31.1±10	BB	40	20, 30, 40, 50, 60%MVC	5	0.1-3000	1
Doheny et al. (2008)	12	24.8±2.8	BB,BR,TB	10	10, 20, 30, 40, 50, 60, 70%MVC	8	20-450	2
Kaplanis et al. (2009)	94	5-69	BB	10	10, 30, 50, 70, 100%MVC	5	20-500	3

Table 2. A survey of the experimental conditions in related works about the effect of muscle force on MNF and MDF in chronological order. Note that CF is one of three conflicting cases for muscle force effect; MA is maximum amplitude; FCR is flexor carpi radialis; BL is brachialis; FL is frontalis; CS is corrugator supercilii; ED is extensor digitorum; TZ is trapezius; TB is triceps brachii; AN is anconeus.

There are several possible reasons for the conflicting results presented above.

Firstly, the different muscles studied have the different muscle fibre composition and distribution, and also the different tissue filter effects (Farina et al., 2002). The EMG power spectrum can be changed by both of which. Moreover, the difference of subject gender can produce the differences in fibre diameters and types (Sabbahi et al., 1981). Hence, the difference in the type and distribution of muscle fibres should be one of the major reasons, although the conflicting results exist in the same muscle i.e. the biceps brachii.

Secondly, the electrode locations over the muscle are different in the experiments. Komi and Viitasalo (1976) mentioned that MNF increase with muscle force levels unless the electrodes were located over the motor point area.

Thirdly, the inter-electrode distance (ID) of the bipolar surface electrodes may be the possible reason for the conflicting results. However, based on the observation throughout Table 2, the different inter-electrode distances are also found in the same case (all cases).

Fourthly, Bilodeau et al. (1992) found the different results between two genders for MDF but not for MNF. The difference in skinfold layer is the main contributor for the differences between two genders in that study. On the other hand, Kaplanis et al. (2009) found that no significant differences exist between values based on gender and age.

Other possible reasons are the limited and different number of subjects (i.e. 4–94 subjects), the level of force exhibited (i.e. %MVC or weight in kg), the range of joint angle exhibited (i.e. 0-150 degrees of extension), the difference in recording time (i.e. 1–30s), the existence of fatigue that resulting from the longer recording times (Lariviere et al., 2001), and the method of statistical analysis used.

To confirm the effect of muscle force on MNF and MDF, the relationship between MNF (and also MDF) and muscle force level was re-evaluated by the new EMG data (Phinyomark et al., 2012c). Figs. 1(a), 1(c) and 1(e) illustrate the relationship between muscle force level and MNF at the constant angle, while Figs. 1(b), 1(d) and 1(f) display the relationship between muscle load level and MDF at the same condition.

Three conflicting cases were found in our experiments for the effect of muscle force on MNF and MDF. The results are the subject-dependent. It is similar as the three conflicting cases which were found in the literature. To answer the question "why's the subject-dependent?", several related anthropometric variables obtained from the volunteers should be intended to find the possible reasons (Phinyomark et al., 2012c). The preliminary study showed that a number of anthropometric variables have a correlation with the conflicting results, such as standing height, hand breadth, body mass, and forward grip reach.

In order to modify MNF and MDF to have the consistent results (the same case), a modification of traditional MNF and MDF should be done. In one of our previous works (Thongpanja et al., 2010), we found that if a concept of using consecutive fast Fourier transform (FFT) is used instead of using a whole signal FFT, a certain relationship between MNF (and MDF) and muscle force level (the third case) can be found in the middle range of consecutive feature series for all trials and subjects, as an example is shown in Fig. 2. This is not found for traditional MNF and MDF. This finding can be applied for the EMG signals recorded from the biceps brachii (Thongpanja et al., 2010, 2011) and also the flexor pollicis longus (Thongpanja et al., 2012). To easily observe and use in applications, five statistical variables consisting mean, median, variance, the RMS and kurtosis are used to apply with the selected efficient range of consecutive feature series. The results showed that the consistent results exist across the subjects (subject-independent) by applying mean and median variables (Thongpanja et al., 2011, 2013). The optimization of such techniques can be found more details in Thongpanja et al. (2013).

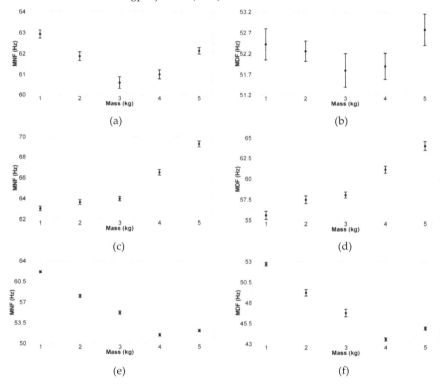

Figure 1. (a, c, e) MNF and (b, d, f) MDF of EMG signals recorded at a constant joint angle (90°) as a function of muscle force (1-5 kg) for three subjects. (a-b) the first case in muscle force effect or CF1 (c-d) the second case in muscle force effect or CF2 (e-f) the third case in muscle force effect or CF3. The error bars shown are given by the standard deviation of the mean value.

5. Effect of muscle geometry on mean and median frequencies

Muscle geometry is another main factor that does significantly affect MNF and MDF. Generally, the effect of muscle geometry including electrode configuration, fibre diameter and subcutaneous tissue thickness has been evaluated by the resulting from changes in joint

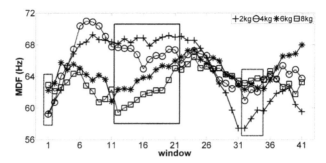

Figure 2. The consecutive MDF feature series computed from the EMG signals recorded from the biceps brachii during dynamic muscle contractions (0-150 degrees of extension). Four load levels are applied: 2, 4, 6 and 8 kg. The FFT is computed using the window size of 512 samples and window overlapping of 64 samples. Note that the second case exists in the beginning and the end ranges (the dashed line boxes) and the third case exists in the middle range (the solid line box).

angle or muscle length (Merletti et al., 1999). Changing in such factors can vary producing a time-varying EMG spectrum. In the literature, two different cases exist for the effect of muscle geometry on MNF and MDF.

In the first case (CG1), MNF and MDF are unaffected by changes in joint angle or muscle length (Sato, 1976). A number of the studies showed no significant change in the power spectrum of EMG signals acquired from the biceps brachii under constant load while joint angle varied. It is also found for the EMG signals recorded from the trapezius, deltoid and the infraspinatus (Gerdle et al., 1988).

In the second case (CG2), MNF (and MDF) increases as muscle length or joint angle (degrees of extension) decreases (Inbar et al., 1987; Shankar et al., 1989). This case exists in most of the studies for EMG signals acquired from the biceps brachii (Cechetto et al., 2001; Doheny et al., 2008; Moritani et al., 1988; Okada, 1987; Potvin, 1997), and is also found for EMG signals acquired from other muscles, such as the tibialis anterior (Merletti et al., 1993), the brachioradialis (Doheny et al., 2008), and the triceps brachii (Doheny et al., 2008; Okada, 1987). The second case, however, is found frequently in the recent studies compared to the first case.

The experimental conditions for several studies are summarized in Table 3. The difference in the experimental conditions may be the reasons for the conflicting results presented in the literature.

Firstly, muscle types and electrode locations over the muscle are different in the experiments. Doheny et al. (2008) mentioned that this factor is one of the reasons for the second case effect. However, the conflicting results are also found in the same muscle i.e. the biceps brachii.

Secondly, Cechetto et al. (2001) proposed that the inter-electrode distance (ID) may be the possible reason for the conflicting results. However, based on the observation through Table 3, three different inter-electrode distances (10, 30 and 40 mm) are found in the same case (the second case).

Thirdly, it can be observed that the frequency band of EMG signals does not affect MNF and MDF.

Reference	N	Age	Muscle	ID	Force levels	Joint angles	Filter	CG
Gerdle et al. (1988)	23	20-30	TZ,DT, IF,BB	-	-	45º, 65º, 90º	-	1
Moritani et al. (1988)	12	-	BB	-	-	30º-150º	-	2
Merletti et al. (1993)	10	-	TA	-	-	0º, 15º, 30º, 45º	-	2
Potvin (1997)	15	24±3	BB	30	7kg	0º-140º	15-450	2
Cechetto et al. (2001)	12	31.1±10	BB	40	20, 30, 40, 50, 60%MVC	50º, 70º, 90º, 110º, 130º	0.1-3000	2
Doheny et al. (2008)	12	24.8±2.8	BB,BR, TB	10	10, 20, 30, 40, 50, 60, 70%MVC	45º, 60º, 75º, 90º, 105º, 120º	20-450	2

Table 3. A survey of the experimental conditions in related works about the effect of muscle geometry (joint angle) on MNF and MDF in chronological order. Note that CF is one of the two conflicting cases for the muscle geometry effect; DT is Deltoid; IF is infraspinatus.

Due to the incompleteness of captured information in the literature, in future study, a request to complete all interested information to the first author or the corresponding author should be done.

As the possible reasons mentioned above that are inconclusive, the main reason for the conflicting results should be the changes of muscle force with the muscle length. The same weight was used at all angles in most of the studies, therefore the changes in MNF and MDF were not due to changes in the muscle length, or joint angle, only but also to changes in the muscle force. In future work, EMG signals should be measured from the muscle under a constant force (varying loads) while joint angles varied.

To confirm the effect of muscle geometry on MNF and MDF, the relationship between MNF (and also MDF) and elbow joint angle was re-evaluated by the similar EMG data as used in Section 4. Figs. 3(a), 3(c) and 3(e) illustrate the relationship between joint angle and MNF at the constant load, while Figs. 3(b), 3(d) and 3(f) display the relationship between joint angle and MDF at the same condition.

Three conflicting cases were found in our experiments for the effect of elbow joint angle on MNF and MDF. The results are the subject-dependent. It is similar as the three conflicting cases which were found in the effect of muscle force on MNF and MDF. In the third case or CG3, MNF (and MDF) increases as muscle length or joint angle (degrees of flexion) increases, as can be observed in Figs. 3(e) and 3(f). In future work, several related anthropometric variables obtained from the volunteers should be intended to find the possible reasons, as mentioned in Section 4.

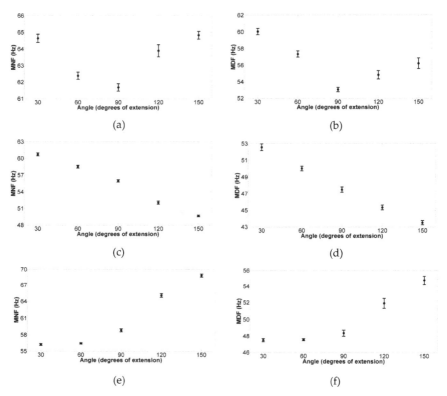

Figure 3. (a, c, e) MNF and (b, d, f) MDF of EMG signals recorded at a constant muscle force (3 kg) as a function of elbow joint angles (30-150 degrees of extension) for three subjects. (a-b) the first case in muscle geometry effect or CG1 (c-d) the second case in muscle geometry effect or CG2 (e-f) the third case in muscle geometry effect or CG3. The error bars shown are given by the standard deviation of the mean value.

In order to modify MNF and MDF to have the consistent results (the same case), a modification of traditional MNF and MDF should be done. Figs. 4(a) and 4(b) show the sample in time-domain of EMG signals measured at the same constant force level with the elbow joint angles at 30º and 150º of extension, respectively. It was found that at narrow elbow joint angles, i.e. 30º of extension, the distribution of positive and negative amplitudes is asymmetry, but at wide elbow joint angles, i.e. 150º of extension, the distribution of positive and negative amplitude is symmetry. The power spectrum of each of the samples is respectively shown in Figs. 4(c) and 4(d). Based on the observation of the distribution, if the EMG signal is normalized by setting the highest value to 1 and the lowest value to -1 for an asymmetric signal, the EMG baseline should be shifted away from the true zero line, as can be observed in Fig. 5(a). On the other hand, the EMG baseline should not be shifted away from the true zero line in the case of normalized symmetric signal, as can be observed in Fig. 5(b). Hence, the values of MNF and MDF that are calculated from the normalized EMG signals measured at the narrow joint angles should decrease, while the values of MNF and MDF that are computed from the normalized EMG signals measured at wide joint angles should be same as the old one. It can be observed throughout Figs. 5(c) and 5(d). As a result, the consistent results should exist across the subjects (subject-independent). The consistent case is the second case. In future work, the evaluation of this finding should be done with the large EMG data set.

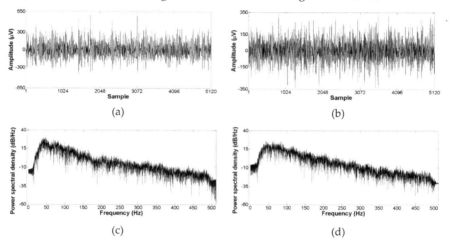

Figure 4. Samples of raw EMG signals recorded from the biceps brachii at (a) 30º and (b) 150º of extension in time-domain, and their power spectrum at (c) 30º and (d) 150º of extension. Note that a constant force (3kg) is performed for each angle.

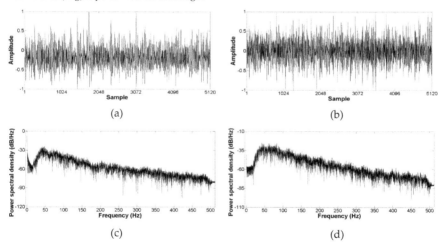

Figure 5. Samples of normalized EMG signals recorded from the biceps brachii at (a) 30º and (b) 150º of extension in time-domain, and their power spectrum at (c) 30º and (d) 150º of extension. Note that a constant force (3kg) is performed for each angle.

6. EMG pattern classification using mean and median frequencies

EMG pattern classification is applied in several potential applications, particularly in the engineering context. The multifunction myoelectric control system (MMCS) is a main engineering application (Oskoei & Hu, 2007; Zecca et al., 2002) consisting the control of prosthesis, industrial robot arms, electric wheelchairs, virtual keyboard and virtual mouse. To be successful in the classification of EMG signals, three main cascaded modules should be carefully considered: data-preprocessing, feature extraction, and classification methods, especially the selection of feature extraction methods (Boostani & Moradi, 2003; Phinyomark et al., 2012a).

Three criteria: maximum class separability, robustness and complexity, have been suggested and generally used to evaluate the EMG features for MMCS. Time-domain features have been usually used to make an optimal feature vector. However, only one feature per EMG channel is obtained from most of the frequency-domain methods (Boostani & Moradi, 2003), and their discriminant patterns in feature space are different from that of time-domain features (Phinyomark et al., 2012a). For a more powerful feature vector, an optimal frequency-domain feature should be combined with other successful time-domain features, such as the waveform length or WL (Oskoei & Hu, 2008), the RMS (Phinyomark et al., 2010), and the Willison amplitude or WAMP (Phinyomark et al., 2011).

First, the classification performance of the MNF and MDF features is discussed. Both features have the similar discriminant patterns, as can be observed from the scatter plots in Figs. 6(a) and 6(b). However, the MNF feature showed (a bit) better performance in class separation than the MDF feature. This can be confirmed by the classification accuracy obtained from the linear discriminant (LD) classifier. Mean and standard deviation of the classification accuracy obtained from MNF and MDF are 75.56±11.8% and 70.54±10.4%, respectively (Phinyomark et al., 2012a). Such classification accuracies are computed based on the classification of six upper-limb movements (hand open or HO, hand close or HC, wrist extension or WE, wrist flexion or WF, forearm pronation or FP, and forearm supination or FS) and five EMG channels (the extensor carpi radialis longus, the extensor carpi ulnaris, the extensor digitorum communis, the flexor carpi radialis, and the biceps brachii) from twenty healthy subjects (ten men and ten women).

For other frequency-domain features, five features consisting TTP, MNP, SM1, SM2 and SM3 have the same discriminant patterns in feature space as features in time-domain i.e. the RMS and the WL (Phinyomark et al., 2012a). Therefore, these features are not recommended to be one of the optimal features due to their higher computational cost. Moreover, the discriminant pattern of PSR is an inverse case of MNF and MDF, but the classification accuracy of PSR is less than that of MNF and MDF.

On the other hand, three features consisting PKF, VCF, and FR have the different discriminant patterns by comparing with MNF, MDF, and also time-domain features. The classification accuracies obtained from the classifier of PKF and VCF are very low (<50%), while the classification accuracy of FR (69.81%) is a bit less than that of MNF and MDF (Phinyomark et al., 2012a). Based on the results mentioned above, it can be concluded that MNF is an optimal frequency-domain feature for the EMG pattern classification.

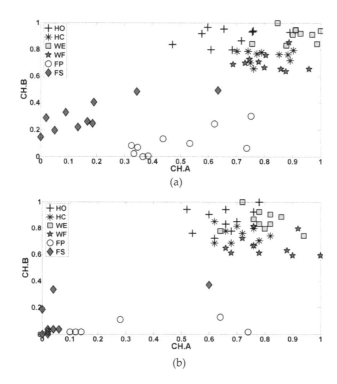

Figure 6. Scatter plots of (a) MNF and (b) MDF for 2 EMG channels (CH.A and CH.B) and 6 upper-limb movements (HO, HC, WE, WF, FP and FS) of a healthy subject. Note that CH.A is flexor carpi radialis muscle; CH.B is extensor carpi radialis longus muscle.

Further, in order to increase the robustness property of the MNF and MDF features, a modification of the MNF and MDF methods was proposed in one of our previous works (Phinyomark et al., 2009). The statistical variables (mean and median) were applied to the amplitude spectrum instead of the power spectrum, as used in the traditional methods, because the variation of the amplitude spectrum is less than that of the power spectrum. As a result, the variation of the modified MNF and MDF features is less than that of the traditional MNF and MDF features. These findings are confirmed using the real EMG data as presented in Phinyomark et al. (2009).

7. Conclusion and future trends

Mean frequency (MNF) and median frequency (MDF) are two useful and popular frequency-domain features for electromyography analysis both in clinical and engineering applications. MNF and MDF are frequently used as the gold standard tool to detect fatigue in the target muscles using EMG signals. The effectiveness of MNF and MDF under many experimental conditions is presented and confirmed in this chapter, although the effects of muscle force and muscle geometry on MNF and MDF are inconclusive. However, the possible reasons for the conflicting results in both effects have been described and discussed in detail together with the possible techniques to make the consistent results for MNF and MDF with the both effects, as mentioned in the following.

- For the effect of muscle force, the selection of time-dependent MNF and MDF should be applied to the raw EMG data. As a result, MNF and MDF should increase as the muscle force or load increases.
- For the effect of muscle geometry or joint angle, the normalization technique should be applied to the raw EMG data. As a result, MNF and MDF should increase as the muscle length or joint angle (degrees of extension) decreases.

However, the question remains whether the conflicting results, i.e. subject dependent, are found for the effect of both muscle force and muscle geometry on MNF and MDF. To address this question, two further works should be investigated: (1) finding the correlation between related anthropometric variables obtained from the subjects and MNF (or MDF), and (2) requesting all interested information to complete all components in Tables 2 and 3, and finding the possible reasons from the complete experimental conditions.

In total, MNF and MDF features extracted from the EMG signal are the optimal variables to identify muscle fatigue, particularly for static muscle contraction. However, for dynamic muscle contraction, applying instantaneous MNF and MDF are recommended.

The recommendations above can be useful to apply for most electromyography applications, such as human-computer interaction (HCI), ergonomics, occupational therapy and sport science. In addition, applying both techniques can make the MNF and MDF features to be the universal indices than can identify all factors including muscle force, muscle geometry, and muscle fatigue.

Author details

Angkoon Phinyomark, Sirinee Thongpanja, Pornchai Phukpattaranont
and Chusak Limsakul
Department of Electrical Engineering, Prince of Songkla University, Songkhla, Thailand

Huosheng Hu
*School of Computer Science & Electronic Engineering, University of Essex, Colchester,
United Kingdom*

8. References

Allison, G. T. & Fujiwara, T. (2002). The Relationship between EMG Median Frequency and Low Frequency Band Amplitude Changes at Different Levels of Muscle Capacity. *Clinical Biomechanics*, Vol.17, No.6, pp. 464-469, ISSN 0268-0033

Al-Mulla, M. R.; Sepulveda, F. and Colley, M. (2011). A Review of Non-invasive Techniques to Detect and Predict localised Muscle Fatigue. *Sensors*, Vol.11, No.4, pp. 3545-3594, ISSN 1424-8220

Al-Mulla, M. R.; Sepulveda, F. and Colley, M. (2012b). sEMG Techniques to Detect and Predict Localised Muscle Fatigue, In: *EMG Methods for Evaluating Muscle and Nerve Function*, Mark Schwartz, pp. 157-186, InTech, ISBN 978-953-307-793-2, Rijeka, Croatia

Arnall, F. A.; Koumantakis, G. A.; Oldham, J. A. & Cooper, R. G. (2002). Between-days Reliability of Electromyographic Measures of Paraspinal Muscle Fatigue at 40, 50 and 60% Levels of Maximal Voluntary Contractile Force. *Clinical Rehabilitation*, Vol.16, No.7, pp. 761-771, ISSN 0269-2155

Balasubramanian, V.; Dutt, A. & Rai, S. (2011). Analysis of Muscle Fatigue in Helicopter Pilots. *Applied Ergonomics*, Vol.42, No.6, pp. 913-918, ISSN 0003-6870

Balestra, G.; Knaflitz, M. & Merletti, R. (1988). Comparison between Myoelectric Signal Mean and Median Frequency Estimated. *Proceedings of EMBC 1988 Annual International Conference of the IEEE Engineering in Medicine and Biology Society*, pp. 1708-1709, ISBN 0-7803-0785-2, New Orleans, LA, USA, November 4-7, 1988

Bilodeau, M.; Arsenault, A. B.; Gravel, D. & Bourbonnais, D. (1991). EMG Power Spectra of Elbow Extensors during Ramp and Step Isometric Contractions. *European Journal of Applied Physiology and Occupational Physiology*, Vol.63, No.1, pp. 24-28, ISSN 0301-5548

Bilodeau, M.; Arsenault, A. B.; Gravel, D. & Bourbonnais, D. (1992). Influence of Gender on the EMG Power Spectrum during an Increasing Force Level. *Journal of Electromyography and Kinesiology*, Vol.2, No.3, pp. 121-129, ISSN 1050-6411

Bilodeau, M.; Schindler-Ivens, S.; Williams, D. M.; Chandran, R. & Sharma, S. S. (2003). EMG Frequency Content Changes with Increasing Force and during Fatigue in the Quadriceps Femoris Muscle of Men and Women. *Journal of Electromyography and Kinesiology*, Vol.13, No.1, pp. 83-92, ISSN 1050-6411

Bonato, P.; Roy, S. H.; Knaflitz, M. & De Luca, C. J. (2001). Time Frequency Parameters of the Surface Myoelectric Signal for Assessing Muscle Fatigue during Cyclic Dynamic Contractions. *IEEE Transactions on Biomedical Engineering*, Vol.48, No.7, pp. 745-753, ISSN 0018-9294

Boostani, R. & Moradi, M. H. (2003). Evaluation of the Forearm EMG Signal Features for the Control of a Prosthetic Hand. *Physiological Measurement*, Vol.24, No.2, pp. 309-319, ISSN 0967-3334

Cechetto, A. D.; Parker, P. A. & Scott, R. N. (2001). The Effects of Four Time-varying Factors on the Mean Frequency of a Myoelectric Signal. *Journal of Electromyography and Kinesiology*, Vol.11, No.5, pp. 347-354, ISSN 1050-6411

Cifrek, M.; Medved, V.; Tonković, S. & Ostojić, S. (2009). Surface EMG based Muscle Fatigue Evaluation in Biomechanics. *Clinical Biomechanics*, Vol.24, No.4, pp. 327-340, ISSN 0268-0033

Cifrek, M.; Tonković, S. & Medved, V. (2000). Measurement and Analysis of Surface Myoelectric Signals during Fatigued Cyclic Dynamic Contractions. *Measurement*, Vol.27, No.2, pp. 85-92, ISSN 0263-2241

Chaffin, D. B. (1973). Localized Muscle Fatigue-definition and Measurement. *Journal of Occupational Medicine*, Vol.15, No.4, pp. 346-354, ISSN 0096-1736

Clancy, E. A.; Farina, D. & Merletti, R. (2005). Cross-comparison of Time- and Frequency-domain Methods for Monitoring the Myoelectric Signal during a Cyclic, Force-varying, Fatiguing Hand-grip Task. *Journal of Electromyography and Kinesiology*, Vol.15, No.3, pp. 256-265, ISSN 1050-6411

De Luca, C. J. (1979). Physiology and Mathematics of Myoelectric Signals. *IEEE Transactions on Biomedical Engineering*, Vol.26, No.6, pp. 313-325, ISSN 0018-9294

De Luca, C. J. (1984). Myoelectric Manifestations of Localized Muscular Fatigue in Humans. *Critical Reviews in Biomedical Engineering*, Vol.11, No.4, pp. 251-279, ISSN 0278-940X

Doheny, E. P.; Lowery, M. M.; FitzPatrick, D. P. & O'Malley, M. J. (2008). Effect of Elbow Joint Angle on Force–EMG Relationships in Human Elbow Flexor and Extensor Muscles. *Journal of Electromyography and Kinesiology*, Vol.18, No.5, pp. 760-770, ISSN 1050-6411

Du, S. & Vuskovic, M. (2004). Temporal vs. Spectral Approach to Feature Extraction from Prehensile EMG Signals. *Proceedings of IRI 2004 IEEE International Conference on Information Reuse and Integration*, pp. 344-350, ISBN 0-7803-8819-4, Las Vegas, NV, USA, November 8-10, 2004

Englehart, K. B. & Parker, P. A. (1994). Single Motor Unit Myoelectric Signal Analysis with Nonstationary Data. *IEEE Transactions on Biomedical Engineering*, Vol.41, No.2, pp. 168-180, ISSN 0018-9294

Farina, D.; Fosci, M. & Merletti, R. (2002). Motor Unit Recruitment Strategies Investigated by Surface EMG Variables. *Journal of Applied Physiology*, Vol.92, No.1, pp. 235-247, ISSN 8750-7587

Farina, D. & Merletti, R. (2000). Comparison of Algorithms for Estimation of EMG Variables during Voluntary Isometric Contractions. *Journal of Electromyography and Kinesiology*, Vol.10, No.5, pp. 337-349, ISSN 1050-6411

Gander, R. E. & Hudgins, R. E. (1985). Power Spectral Density of the Surface Myoelectric Signal of the Biceps Brachii as a Function of Static Load. *Electromyography and Clinical Neurophysiology*, Vol.25, No.7-8, pp. 469-478, ISSN 0301-150X

Georgakis, A., Stergioulas, L. K. & Giakas, G. (2003). Fatigue Analysis of the Surface EMG Signal in Isometric Constant Force Contractions Using the Averaged Instantaneous Frequency. *IEEE Transactions on Biomedical Engineering*, Vol.50, No.2, pp. 262-265, ISSN 0018-9294

Gerdle, B.; Eriksson, N. E.; Brundin, L. & Edstrom, M. (1988). Surface EMG Recordings during Maximum Static Shoulder Forward Flexion in Different Positions. *European Journal of Applied Physiology and Occupational Physiology*, Vol.57, No.4, pp. 415-419, ISSN 0301-5548

Gerdle, B.; Eriksson, N. E. & Brundin, L. (1990). The Behaviour of Mean Power Frequency of the Surface Electromyogram in Biceps Brachii with Increasing Force and during Fatigue. With Special regard to the Electrode Distance. *Electromyography and Clinical Neurophysiology*, Vol.30, No.8, pp. 483-489, ISSN 0301-150X

Hagberg, M. & Ericsson, B. E. (1982). Myoelectric Power Spectrum Dependence on Muscular Contraction Level of Elbow Flexors. *European Journal of Applied Physiology and Occupational Physiology*, Vol.48, No.2, pp. 147-156, ISSN 0301-5548

Hagberg, C. & Hagberg, M. (1989). Surface EMG Amplitude and Frequency Dependence on Exerted Force for the Upper Trapezius Muscle: A Comparison between Right and Left Sides. *European Journal of Applied Physiology and Occupational Physiology*, Vol.58, No.6, pp. 641-645, ISSN 0301-5548

Han, J. -S.; Song, W. -K.; Kim, J. -S.; Bang, W. -C.; Lee, H. & Bien, Z. (2000). New EMG Pattern Recognition Based on Soft Computing Techniques and its Application to Control a Rehabilitation Robotic Arm. *Proceedings of IIZUKA 2000 6th International Conference on Soft Computing*, pp. 890-897, Fukuoka, Japan, October 1-4, 2000

Hautier, C. A.; Arsac, L. M.; Deghdegh, K.; Souquet, J.; Belli, A. & Lacour, J. R. (2000). Influence of Fatigue on EMG/Force Ratio and Cocontraction in Cycling. *Medicine and Science in Sports and Exercise*, Vol.32, No.4, pp. 839-843, ISSN 0195-9131

Hermens, H. J.; Boon, K. L. & Zilvold, G. (1984). The Clinical Use of Surface EMG. *Electromyography and Clinical Neurophysiology*, Vol.24, No.4, pp. 243-265, ISSN 0301-150X

Inbar, G. F.; Allin, J. & Kranz, H. (1987). Surface EMG Spectral Changes with Muscle Length. *Medical and Biological Engineering and Computing*, Vol.25, No.6, pp. 683-689, ISSN 0140-0118

Inbar, G. F.; Allin, J.; Paiss, O. & Kranz, H. (1986). Monitoring Surface EMG Spectral Changes by the Zero Crossing Rate. *Medical and Biological Engineering and Computing*, Vol.24, No.1, pp. 10-18, ISSN 0140-0118

Kalra, C. ; Kumar, D. K. & Arjunan, S. (2012). Age and Gender Related Differences on Surface Electromyogram During Various Levels of Contraction. *Journal of Medical and Biological Engineering*, in press, ISSN 1609-0985

Kaplanis, P. A.; Pattichis, C. S.; Hadjileontiadis, L. J. & Roberts, V. C. (2009). Surface EMG Analysis on Normal Subjects Based on Isometric Voluntary Contraction. *Journal of Electromyography and Kinesiology*, Vol.19, No.1, pp. 157-171, ISSN 1050-6411

Karlsson, S.; Yu, J. & Akay, M. (2000). Time-frequency Analysis of Myoelectric Signals during Dynamic Contractions: A Comparative Study. *IEEE Transactions on Biomedical Engineering*, Vol.47, No.2, pp. 228-238, ISSN 0018-9294

Knaflitz, M. and Bonato, P. (1999). Time-frequency Methods Applied to Muscle Fatigue Assessment during Dynamic Contractions. *Journal of Electromyography and Kinesiology*, Vol.9, No.5, pp. 337-350, ISSN 1050-6411

Knaflitz, M.; Merletti, R. & De Luca, C. J. (1990). Inference of Motor Unit Recruitment Order in Voluntary and Electrically Elicited Contractions. *Journal of Applied Physiology*, Vol.68, No.4, pp. 1657-1667, ISSN 8750-7587

Lariviere, C.; Arsenault, A. B.; Gravel, D.; Gagnon, D. & Loisel, P. (2001). Median Frequency of the Electromyographic Signal: Effect of Time-window Location on Brief Step Contractions. *Journal of Electromyography and Kinesiology*, Vol.11, No.1, pp. 65-71, ISSN 1050-6411

Leunkeu, A. N.; Keefer, D. J.; Imed, M. & Ahmaidi, S. (2010). Electromyographic (EMG) Analysis of Quadriceps Muscle Fatigue in Children with Cerebral Palsy during a Sustained Isometric Contraction. *Journal of Child Neurology*, Vol.25, No.3, pp. 287-293, ISSN 0883-0738

MacIsaac, D.; Parker, P. A. & Scott, R. N. (2001). The Short-time Fourier Transform and Muscle Fatigue Assessment in Dynamic Contractions. *Journal of Electromyography and Kinesiology*, Vol.11, No.6, pp. 439-449, ISSN 1050-6411

Mannion, A. F. & Dolan, P. (1996). Relationship between Myoelectric and Mechanical Manifestations of Fatigue in the Quadriceps Femoris Muscle Group. *European Journal of Applied Physiology and Occupational Physiology*, Vol.74, No., pp. 411-419, ISSN 0301-5548

Masuda, K.; Masuda, T.; Sadoyama, T.; Mitsuharu, I. & Katsuta, S. (1999). Changes in Surface EMG Parameters during Static and Dynamic Fatiguing Contractions. *Journal of Electromyography and Kinesiology*, Vol.9, No.1, pp. 39-46, ISSN 1050-6411

Merletti, R.; Lo Conte, L. R.; Avignone, E. & Guglielminotti, P. (1999). Modeling of Surface Myoelectric Signals - Part I : Model Implementation. *IEEE Transactions on Biomedical Engineering*, Vol.46, No.7, pp. 810-820, ISSN 0018-9294

Merletti, R.; Lo Conte, L. R.; Cisari, C. & Massazza, U. (1993). Effect of Ankle Joint Position on Electrically Evoked Surface Myoelectric Signals of the Tibialis Anterior Muscle. *Archives of Physical Medicine and Rehabilitation*, Vol.74, No.5, pp. 501-506, ISSN 0003-9993

Merletti, R. & Parker, P. (2004). *ELECTROMYOGRAPHY Physiology, Engineering, and Noninvasive Applications*, John Wiley & Sons, ISBN 0-471-67580-6, USA

Merletti, R. & Roy, S. (1996). Myoelectric and Mechanical Manifestations of Muscle Fatigue in Voluntary Contractions. *Journal of Orthopaedic and Sports Physical Therapy*, Vol.24, No.6, pp. 342-353, ISSN 0190-6011

Merletti, R.; Sabbahi, M. A. & De Luca, C. J. (1984). Median Frequency of the Myoelectric Signal: Effects of Muscle Ischemia and Cooling. *European Journal of Applied Physiology and Occupational Physiology*, Vol.52, No.3, pp. 258-265, ISSN 0301-5548

Moritani, T.; Muramatsu, S. & Muro, M. (1988). Activity of Motor Units during Concentric and Eccentric Contractions. *American Journal of Physical Medicine*, Vol.66, No.6, pp. 338-350, ISSN 0002-9491

Moritani, T. & Muro, M. (1987). Motor Unit Activity and Surface Electromyogram Power Spectrum during Increasing Force of Contraction. *European Journal of Applied Physiology and Occupational Physiology*, Vol.56, No.3, pp. 260-265, ISSN 0301-5548

Muro, M. ; Nagata, A.; Murakami, K. & Moritani, T. (1982). Surface EMG Power Spectral Analysis of Neuromuscular Disorders during Isometric and Isotonic Contraction. *American Journal of Physical Medicine*, Vol.61, No.5, pp. 244-254, ISSN 0894-9115

Okada, M. (1987). Effect of Muscle Length on Surface EMG Wave Forms in Isometric Contractions. *European Journal of Applied Physiology and Occupational Physiology*, Vol.56, No.4, pp. 482-486, ISSN 1439-6319

Oskoei, M. A. & Hu, H. (2006). GA-based Feature Subset Selection for Myoelectric Classification. *Proceedings of ROBIO 2006 IEEE International Conference on Robotics and Biomimetics*, pp. 1465-1470, ISBN 1-4244-0570-X, Kunming, China, December 17-20, 2006

Oskoei, M. A. & Hu, H. (2007). Myoelectric Control Systems—A Survey. *Biomedical Signal Processing and Control*, Vol.2, No.4, pp. 275-294, ISSN 1746-8094

Oskoei, M. A. & Hu, H. (2008). Support Vector Machine based Classification Scheme for Myoelectric Control Applied to Upper Limb. *IEEE Transactions on Biomedical Engineering*, Vol.55, No.8, pp. 1956-1965, ISSN 0018-9294

Oskoei, M. A.; Hu, H. & Gan, J. Q. (2008). Manifestation of Fatigue in Myoelectric Signals of Dynamic Contractions Produced during Playing PC Games. *Proceedings of EMBS 2008 30th Annual International Conference of the IEEE Engineering in Medicine and Biology Society*, pp. 315-318, ISBN 978-1-4244-1814-5, Vancouver, BC, Canada, August 20-25, 2008

Petrofsky, J. S.; Glaser, R. M.; Philips, C. A.; Lind, A. R. & Williams, C. (1982). Evaluation of Amplitude and Frequency Components of the Surface EMG as an Index of Muscle Fatigue. *Ergonomics*, Vol.25, No.3, pp. 213-223, ISSN 0014-0139

Petrofsky, J. S. & Lind, A. R. (1980a). Frequency Analysis of the Surface Electromyogram during Sustained Isometric Contractions. *European Journal of Applied Physiology and Occupational Physiology*, Vol.43, No.2, pp. 173-182, ISSN 0301-5548

Petrofsky, J. S. & Lind, A. R. (1980b). The Influence of Temperature on the Amplitude and Frequency Components of the EMG during Brief and Sustained Isometric Contractions. *European Journal of Applied Physiology and Occupational Physiology*, Vol.44, No.2, pp. 189-200, ISSN 0301-5548

Phinyomark, A.; Limsakul, C. & Phukpattaranont, P. (2009). A Novel Feature Extraction for Robust EMG Pattern Recognition. *Journal of Computing*, Vol.1, No.1, pp. 71-80, ISSN 2151-9617

Phinyomark, A.; Hirunviriya, S.; Phukpattaranont, P. & Limsakul, C. (2010). Evaluation of EMG Feature Extraction for Hand Movement Recognition Based on Euclidean Distance and Standard Deviation. *Proceedings of ECTI-CON 2010 7th International Conference on Electrical Engineering/Electronics, Computer, Telecommunications and Information Technology*, pp. 856-860, ISBN 978-1-4244-5606-2, Chiang Mai, Thailand, May 19-21, 2010

Phinyomark, A.; Hirunviriya, S.; Nuidod, A.; Phukpattaranont, P. & Limsakul, C. (2011). Evaluation of EMG Feature Extraction for Movement Control of Upper Limb Prostheses Based on Class Separation Index. *IFMBE Proceedings*, Vol. 35, Part 8, pp. 750-754, ISSN 1680-0737

Phinyomark, A.; Phukpattaranont, P. & Limsakul, C. (2012a). Feature Reduction and Selection for EMG Signal Classification. *Expert Systems with Applications*, Vol.39, No.8, pp. 7420-7431, ISSN 0957-4174

Phinyomark, A.; Phukpattaranont, P. & Limsakul, C. (2012b). The Usefulness of Wavelet Transform to Reduce Noise in the SEMG Signal, In: *EMG Methods for Evaluating Muscle and Nerve Function*, Mark Schwartz, pp. 107-132, InTech, ISBN 978-953-307-793-2, Rijeka, Croatia

Phinyomark, A.; Thongpanja, S.; Phukpattaranont, P. & Limsakul, C. (2012c). Investigation of Conflicting Results of Muscle Force Effect on Mean and Median Frequencies. *Australasian Physical and Engineering Sciences in Medicine*, in submitted, ISSN 0158-9938

Potvin, J. R. (1997). Effects of Muscle Kinematics on Surface EMG Amplitude and Frequency during Fatiguing Dynamic Contractions. *Journal of Applied Physiology*, Vol.82, No.1, pp. 144-151, ISSN 0021-8987

Qingju, Z. & Zhizeng, L. (2006). Wavelet De-noising of Electromyography. *Proceedings of ICMA 2006 IEEE International Conference on Mechatronics Automation*, pp. 1553–1558, ISBN 1-4244-0465-7, Luoyang, Henan, China, June 25-28, 2006

Rainoldi, A.; Galardi, G.; Maderna, L.; Comi, G.; Conte, L. L. & Merletti, R. (1999). Repeatability of Surface EMG Variables during Voluntary Isometric Contraction of the Biceps Brachii Muscle. *Journal of Electromyography and Kinesiology*, Vol.9, No.2, pp. 105-119, ISSN 1050-6411

Ravier, P.; Buttelli, O.; Jennane, R. & Couratier, P. (2005). An EMG Fractal Indicator Having Different Sensitivities to Changes in Force and Muscle Fatigue during Voluntary Static Muscle Contractions. *Journal of Electromyography and Kinesiology*, Vol.15, No.2, pp. 210-221, ISSN 1050-6411

Roy, S. H., Bonato, P. & Knaflitz, M. (1998). EMG Assessment of Back Muscle Function during Cyclical Lifting. *Journal of Electromyography and Kinesiology*, Vol.8, No.4, pp. 233-245, ISSN 1050-6411

Sabbahi, M. A.; Merletti, R.; De Luca, C. J. & Rosenthal, R. G. (1981). How Handiness, Sexa md Force Level Affect the Median Frequency of the Myoelectric Signal. *Proceedings of 1981 4th Annual Conference on Rehabilitation Engineering*, pp. 232-234, Washington, D.C., USA, August 30-September 3, 1981

Sato, H. (1976). Some Factors Affecting the Power Spectra of Surface Electromyograms in Isometric Contractions. *Journal of Anthropology of the Nippon Society*, Vol.84, No.2, pp. 105-113, ISSN 0918-7960

Sato, H. (1982). Functional Characteristics of Human Skeletal Muscle Revealed by Spectral Analysis of the Surface Electromyogram. *Electromyography and Clinical Neurophysiology*, Vol.22, No.6, pp. 459-516, ISSN 0301-150X

Shankar, S.; Gander, R. E. & Brandell, B. R. (1989). Changes in the Myoelectric Signal (MES) Power Spectra during Dynamic Contractions. *Electroencephalography and Clinical Neurophysiology*, Vol.73, No.2, pp. 142-150, ISSN 0013-4694

Soares, F. A.; Salomoni, S. E.; Veneziano, W. H.; De Carvalho, J. L. A.; Nascimento, F. A. D. O.; Pires, K. F. & Da Rocha, A. F. (2011). On the Behavior of Surface Electromyographic Variables during the Menstrual Cycle. *Physiological Measurement*, Vol.32, No.5, pp. 543-557, ISSN 0967-3334

Solomonow, M.; Baten, C.; Smit, J.; Baratta, R.; Hermens, H.; D'Ambrosia, R. & Shoji, H. (1990). Electromyogram Power Spectra Frequencies Associated with Motor Unit Recruitment Strategies. *Journal of Applied Physiology*, Vol.68, No.3, pp. 1177-1185, ISSN 0021-8987

Stulen, F. B. & De Luca, C. J. (1981). Frequency Parameters of the Myoelectric Signal as a Measure of Muscle Conduction Velocity. *IEEE Transactions on Biomedical Engineering*, Vol.28, No.7, pp. 515-523, ISSN 0018-9294

Tavakolan, M.; Xiao, Z. G. & Menon, C. (2011). A Preliminary Investigation Assessing the Viability of Classifying Hand Postures in Seniors. *Biomedical Engineering* Online, Vol.10, No.79, ISSN 1475-925X

Thongpanja, S.; Phinyomark, A.; Phukpattaranont, P. & Limsakul, C. (2010). Time-dependent EMG Power Spectrum Features of Biceps Brachii During Isotonic Exercise. *Journal of Sports Science and Technology*, Vol.10, No.2S, pp. 314-318, ISSN 1513-7201

Thongpanja, S.; Phinyomark, A.; Phukpattaranont, P. & Limsakul, C. (2011). Time-dependent EMG Power Spectrum Parameters of Biceps Brachii During Cyclic Dynamic Contraction. *IFMBE Proceedings*, Vol.35, No.8, pp. 233-236, ISSN 1680-0737

Thongpanja, S.; Phinyomark, A.; Phukpattaranont, P. & Limsakul, C. (2012). A Feasibility Study of Fatigue and Muscle Contraction Indices Based on EMG Time-dependent Spectral Analysis. *Procedia Engineering*, Vol.32, pp. 239-245, ISSN 1877-7058

Thongpanja, S.; Phinyomark, A.; Phukpattaranont, P. & Limsakul, C. (2013). Mean and Median Frequency of EMG Signal to Determine Muscle Force Based on Time-Dependent Power Spectrum. *Electronics and Electrical Engineering*, Vol.129, No.3, ISSN 2029-5731

Van Boxtel, A. & Schomaker, L. R. B. (1984). Influence of Motor Unit Firing Statistics on the Median Frequency of the EMG Power Spectrum. *European Journal of Applied Physiology and Occupational Physiology*, Vol.52, No.2, pp. 207-213, ISSN 0301-5548

Viitasalo, J. T. & Komi, P. V. (1977). Signal Characteristics of EMG during Fatigue. *European Journal of Applied Physiology and Occupational Physiology*, Vol.37, No.2, pp. 111-121, ISSN 0301-5548

Viitasalo, J. T. & Komi, P. V. (1978). Interrelationships of EMG Signal Characteristics at Different Levels of Muscle Tension and during Fatigue. *Electromyography and Clinical Neurophysiology*, Vol.18, No.3-4, pp. 167-178, ISSN 0301-150X

Zaman, S. A.; MacIsaac, D. T. & Parker, P. A. (2011). Repeatability of Surface EMG-based Single Parameter Muscle Fatigue Assessment Strategies in Static and Cyclic Contractions. *Proceedings of EMBC 2011 33rd Annual International Conference of the IEEE Engineering in Medicine and Biology Society*, pp. 3857-3860, ISBN 978-142444121-1, Boston, MA, USA, August 30-September 3, 2011

Zecca, M.; Micera, S.; Carrozza, M. C. & Dario, P. (2002). Control of Multifunctional Prosthetic Hands by Processing the Electromyographic Signal. *Critical Reviews in Biomedical Engineering*, Vol.30, No.4-6, pp. 459-485, ISSN 0278-940X

Zhang, Z. G.; Liu, H. T.; Chan, S. C.; Luk, K. D. & Hu, Y. (2010). Time-dependent Power
     Spectral Density Estimation of Surface Electromyograhy during Isometric Muscle
     Contraction : Methods and Comparisons. *Journal of Electromyography and Kinesiology*,
     Vol.20, No.1, pp. 89-101, ISSN 1050-6411

Feature Extraction Methods for Studying Surface Electromyography and Kinematic Measurements in Parkinson's Disease

Saara M. Rissanen, Markku Kankaanpää,
Mika P. Tarvainen and Pasi A. Karjalainen

Additional information is available at the end of the chapter

1. Introduction

1.1. Parkinson's disease (PD)

Parkinson's disease is a progressive neurodegenerative disease that affects 1 % of people over 60 years of age [9]. In PD, there is a dopaminergic neuronal loss in the substantia nigra in the basal ganglia of the cerebra [48]. It has been observed that the basal ganglia has a specific effect on the temporal organization of motor cortical activity during muscle contractions. In this way, the dysfunction of the basal ganglia may lead to motor symptoms of PD. [37] The primary symptoms of PD include tremor, muscle rigidity and slowness of movements. The diagnosis is based on the presence of the primary symptoms and on the response to medication. [17, 18]. However, the diagnosis can be problematic. Clinicopathological studies from the UK and Canada have shown that the disease is diagnosed incorrectly in about 25 % of patients [48]. The pre-motor period before diagnosis may be long (5–20 years) and at the time of the diagnosis already 50–60 % of the dopaminergic neurons may be lost [22, 38].

Although there is no cure for PD, the symptoms can be relieved reasonably with medication or with the deep brain stimulation (DBS) [17]. The motor impairment, the disease progression and the efficacy of treatment are commonly evaluated subjectively using standardized rating scales such as the Unified Parkinson's disease rating scale (UPDRS) [12, 15]. No objectively measured characteristics and methods are widely used for quantifying motor symptoms of PD [2].

Several objective methods have been proposed for improving the diagnostic accuracy of PD, for enabling earlier diagnosis, and for quantifying the disease severity, progression and the efficacy of treatment. These methods include: kinematic measurements of motor tasks (e.g. finger tapping), testing of olfactory loss, imaging techniques (e.g. magnetic resonance imaging and positron emission tomography), and biochemical tests of blood and cerebrospinal fluid.

However, none of the proposed methods is widely used for PD. The validation of new methods for clinical use takes time. In order to be more sensitive than the traditional methods it is probable that a combination of several methods will be needed for PD. [2, 11, 24]

1.2. Surface electromyography and kinematic measurements in PD

Surface electromyography (EMG) and kinematic measurements are non-invasive and relatively simple and cost-effective methods for quantifying neuromuscular function and movement. Therefore, these methods may be suitable for quantifying objectively the motor impairment in PD and the effects of treatment. A few new technologies based on kinematic sensors have been recently commercialized for measuring motor symptoms of PD. The kinematic measurements provide information about human movements. However, it is possible that surface EMG provides earlier or more direct information about PD than the sole kinematic measures based on movement.

Several studies have analyzed the surface EMG and kinematic signals of PD patients in comparison to the signals of healthy subjects and aimed to correlate the most significant findings with the clinical rating scales. Differences between patients and healthy subjects have been observed in the tremor-EMG coherence [50], in the cortico-muscular coherence [37] and in the muscle activation patterns during limb movements [13, 26, 35]. In the gait characteristics, differences have been observed in the gait speed and stride length, in the arm and leg swing and in the muscle activation patterns of gait [5–7, 36, 43].

Several studies have evaluated effects of PD treatment (medication and DBS) on the basis of EMG and kinematic measurements. It has been observed that the medication and DBS may modify the tremor amplitude, regularity and frequency [4, 41, 42], movement speed [3, 8, 34, 40, 44, 49, 51, 52], joint kinetics and muscle activation during movements [55], EMG burst patterns during movement [34, 51, 52] and the cortico-muscular coherence [25, 37]. There is currently a lot of interest for characterizing EMG and kinematic signals of PD patients. However, many studies have analyzed the EMG signals of PD patients by using conventional amplitude- and spectral based methods. More information about PD could be extracted from the EMG signals by using also more modern methods of signal analysis, by analyzing sets of signal features and by analyzing the signal characteristics also on individual level.

EMG signals are impulse-like waveforms because they consist of motor unit (MU) action potentials. The level of MU synchronization is increased in PD [14, 50], which appears as an increased number of recurring spikes and bursts in the EMG signals. Therefore, there is important information about PD in the morphology of the EMG signal and in the recurring signal patterns. It has been observed that the conventional EMG signal parameters (amplitudes and the mean and median frequencies) are not effective in capturing impulse-like structures [23]. Therefore, more modern methods of signal analysis are needed for analyzing the EMG signals of PD patients.

1.3. Our approach for studying surface EMG and kinematic measurements in PD

In order to extract PD-related information from the surface EMG signals effectively, we proposed specific methods based on signal morphology, nonlinear dynamics and wavelets for analyzing the EMG signals of PD patients in [28–32]. One aim of those studies was to develop objective methods for discriminating between PD patients and healthy subjects on the basis of surface EMG signal morphology [32] and on the basis of simultaneous EMG and acceleration (ACC) recordings during isometric [28] and dynamic muscle contractions [29]. Another aim was to develop methods based on surface EMG and kinematic measurements and analysis for quantifying effects of PD treatment (medication and DBS) on individual level. All of those studies presented an innovative approach, that combines a principal component (PC) -based method with a set of effective signal features, for analyzing the EMG and acceleration signals in PD. In the following sections 2, 3 and 4, we describe the methods that were developed and used for feature extraction and discrimination between subjects in [28–32]. All methods were tested with the measured data. In total, the measurement data from 62 PD patients and 72 healthy subjects were analyzed. The main findings of those studies are also described.

2. Analysis EMG signal morphology in PD

EMG signal is a sum of MU action potentials at a given location and therefore it is an impulse-like waveform. The EMG signals of PD patients are characterized by recurring spikes and bursts (see Figure 1) that are likely caused by the increased level of MU synchronization. Important information about PD is in the EMG signal morphology and in the recurring signal patters.

In [32], the EMG signal morphology of 25 PD patients and 22 healthy subjects was analyzed by using sample histograms and crossing rate (CR) expansions. The analyzed EMG signals were measured during the isometric contraction of biceps brachii (BB) muscles. During the task, subjects were asked to hold their elbows at a 90° angle with their palms up. The measurements were performed by using the ME6000 -biosignal monitor (Mega Electronics Ltd., Kuopio, Finland) and disposable Ag/AgCl electrodes (Medicotest, model M-00-S, Ølstykke, Denmark) in bipolar connection. The sampling rate was 1000 Hz.

Typical EMG signals of one healthy subject and one PD patient are presented in Figure 1. One can observe that the EMG signal of the patient contains recurring EMG bursts while the EMG signal of the healthy subject does not.

2.1. Feature extraction by using sample histograms and CR expansions

Sample histograms were extracted from the scaled (between -1 and 1) EMG signals with 200 bins and the CR expansions from the scaled EMGs as the number of crossings at given threshold levels (201 threshold levels). An example of the sample histogram and the CR expansion for the healthy subject and for the PD patient are presented in Figure 1. One can observe that the sample histogram of the patient is sharper and the CR expansion narrower than those of the healthy subject.

2.2. Discrimination analysis between subjects

The calculated sample histograms and CR expansions of PD patients (with medication on) and healthy subjects were used as high-dimensional feature vectors for discrimination analysis between subjects. The PC-based approach was used for decreasing the dimensionality of the

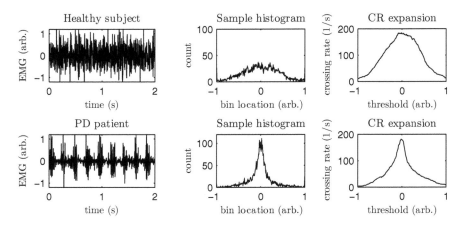

Figure 1. EMG signals of one healthy subject (top) and one PD patient (bottom). The sample histograms and crossing rate expansions of the healthy subject and the PD patient.

feature vectors and the discriminant analysis of subjects was performed in a two-dimensional feature space.

In the PC-based approach [19], each feature vector $z_j \in \mathbb{R}^{N_p}$ is modeled with a linear model

$$z_j = H\theta_j + v_j. \tag{1}$$

In the linear model, $H = [\phi_1 \ \phi_2 \ \cdots \ \phi_K] \in \mathbb{R}^{N_p \times K}$ is the model matrix that contains the basis vectors $\phi_k \in \mathbb{R}^{N_p}$ in its columns. Vector $\theta_j \in \mathbb{R}^K$ contains the model weights and $v_j \in \mathbb{R}^{N_p}$ the model error for the j'th feature vector. The basis vectors ϕ_k are selected to be the eigenvectors of the data correlation matrix

$$R_z = \frac{1}{M} \sum_{j=1}^{M} z_j z_j^T, \tag{2}$$

where M is the total number of feature vectors and $(\cdot)^T$ denotes the transpose. Because the eigenvectors are orthonormal, the least squares solution for the model weights θ_j is of the form

$$\hat{\theta}_j = (H^T H)^{-1} H^T z_j = H^T z_j. \tag{3}$$

These weights are called the principal components. By choosing K ($K < N_p$) eigenvectors corresponding to K largest eigenvalues for modeling, the best K-dimensional orthogonal approximation for the data set is obtained. The PCs are the new uncorrelated features and they can be used for discriminating between subjects in a low-dimensional feature space.

In [32], three feature vectors were formed for each subject: one containing the EMG sample histogram, one containing the CR expansion and one containing both of them (augmented PC approach). Thus, the original dimensionality of the feature vectors was reasonably high ($N_p \geq 200$). The feature vectors of one PD patient and one healthy subject in the augmented

PC approach are illustrated in Figure 2. In addition, the correlation matrix and the three
eigenvectors corresponding to the three largest eigenvalues are presented in the same figure.

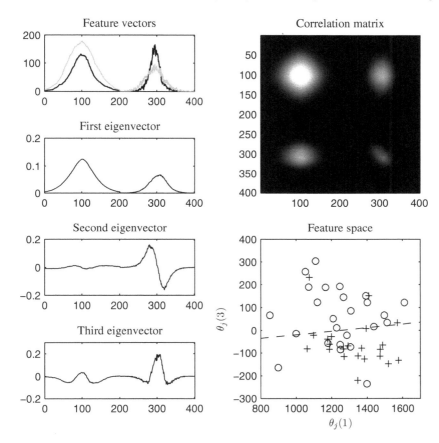

Figure 2. The feature vectors of one PD patient (black) and one healthy subject (gray) in the augmented
PC approach (top left). Three eigenvectors corresponding to the three largest eigenvalues (left). The data
correlation matrix (top right). The third PCs $\theta_j(3)$ with respect to the first PCs $\theta_j(1)$ of 22 healthy subjects
(+) and 25 PD patients (o) (bottom right).

The correlation matrix in Figure 2 contains four white areas with high correlation. The white
area in the top left corner describes correlations between the CR expansion values. The white
area in the bottom right corner describes correlations between the sample histogram values.
The non-diagonal white areas describe cross-correlations between the CR expansion values
and the sample histogram values.

The eigenvectors in Figure 2 can be interpreted as follows:

- The first eigenvector is the best mean-square fit for the feature vectors of all subjects. Thus, it is similar to the mean of all feature vectors. Therefore, the first PC describes the amplitude of the histogram and the CR expansion with respect to the mean of all subjects.

- The second eigenvector is the best mean-square fit for the residual of the first fit. The second eigenvector describes variations in the peaks (modes) of the histograms and CR expansions of all subjects.

- The third eigenvector models variations in the heights and widths of the histograms and CR expansions in the whole data set.

The rest of the eigenvectors contain information about higher frequencies of the data and do not interest us in this case. The biggest differences between patients and healthy subjects were found in the third PC and some differences were observed in the first PC. Therefore, the discrimination between subjects was performed with respect to the third and the first PC.

2.3. Results

A linear discriminant was used in [32] for discriminating between the subjects in the two-dimensional feature space that was spanned by the third and the first PCs. The best discrimination results were obtained by using the augmented PC approach (see results in Figure 2). According to the results, 72 % of PD patients can be discriminated from 86 % of healthy subjects on the basis of EMG signal morphology.

3. Analysis of simultaneous EMG and acceleration recordings in PD

3.1. EMG and acceleration measurements

We analyzed simultaneous EMG and acceleration measurements of PD patients and healthy subjects in [28, 29] and aimed to develop methods for discriminating between the patients and the healthy subjects on the basis of the measured signals. The signals were measured during isometric contraction of BB muscles [28] and during dynamic elbow flexion-extension movements [29].

During the isometric task, the subjects were asked to hold their elbows at a 90° angle with their palms up. During the dynamic task, the subjects were asked to flex and extend their both elbows vertically and freely in two-second cycles with their palms up. Surface EMGs were registered continuously from the BB muscles and the accelerations of forearms simultaneously from the palmar side of subject's wrists. All measurements were performed by using the ME6000 -biosignal monitor (Mega Electronics Ltd., Kuopio, Finland), disposable Ag/AgCl electrodes (Medicotest, model M-00-S, Ølstykke, Denmark) in bipolar connection and tri-axial accelerometers (Meac-x, Mega Electronics Ltd., range ±10 g). Signals were sampled with the rate of 1000 Hz. The resultant of the acceleration was used in the analysis. Low-frequency trends were removed from both signals by using the smoothness priors method [46]. The high-pass cut-off frequencies were 10 Hz for EMG and 2 Hz for acceleration.

Typical EMG and acceleration signals of one PD patient and one healthy subject during the isometric and dynamic task are presented in Figure 3. It is observed in the isometric

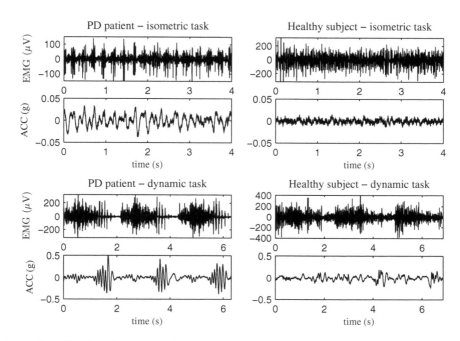

Figure 3. EMG and acceleration recordings of one PD patient (left) and one healthy subject (right) during the isometric and the dynamic task.

recording, that the EMG signal of the PD patient differs from the EMG signal of the healthy subject by containing recurring EMG bursts and the acceleration signal by containing regular high-amplitude oscillation. This oscillation is likely due to the resting and postural tremor. It is observed in the dynamic recording, that the EMG signal of the PD patient is characterized by recurring spikes and the acceleration recording by containing high-amplitude oscillation during the extension phases of the movement. The oscillation in the acceleration signal (which was high-pass-filtered with 2 Hz as cut-off frequency) is likely due to muscle rigidity and kinetic tremor (tremor that occurs during movement). In the flexion phases of the movement, the differences between the patient and the healthy subject are not as pronounced.

3.2. Feature extraction from EMG and acceleration signals

It was observed in [23] and [28, 29] that the conventional amplitude- and spectral-based EMG parameters (root mean square value and median frequency) are not effective in characterizing the EMG signals of PD patients in comparison to the signals of the healthy subjects. Therefore, we extracted a set of other PD characteristic signal features from the isometric [28] and dynamic EMG and acceleration recordings [29]. These parameters are detailed in Table 1 and they were calculated as epoch averages from the isometric EMG and acceleration signals and as time-varying from the dynamic signals.

Task type	Signal features	Notations
Isometric	sample kurtosis of EMG	k_r and k_l
	crossing rate variable of EMG	cr_r and cr_l
	correlation dimension of EMG	$D_{2,r}$ and $D_{2,l}$
	recurrence rate of EMG	$\%REC_r$ and $\%REC_l$
	sample entropy of ACC	$SampEn_r$ and $SampEn_l$
	coherence between EMG and ACC	Coh_r and Coh_l
Dynamic	recurrence rate of EMG	$\%REC_r$ and $\%REC_l$
	cross-recurrence rate of EMG	$\%REC_{r,l}$
	wavelet variable of EMG	$W_{max,r}$ and $W_{max,l}$
	cross-wavelet variable of EMG	$W_{max,rl}$
	power of ACC	$P_{acc,r}$ and $P_{acc,l}$
	sample entropy of ACC	$SampEn_r$ and $SampEn_l$

Table 1. PD characteristic signal features and their notations. The subscripts r and l in the notations stand for the side of the body.

3.2.1. Parameters of surface EMG signal morphology

In [28], we used two parameters (k and cr) for measuring the peakedness of EMG signals. The sample kurtosis was calculated as the fourth centered moment of the time series x (length N):

$$k = \frac{\frac{1}{N} \sum_{i=1}^{N} (x_i - \mu_x)^4}{\sigma_x^4}, \tag{4}$$

where μ_x is the mean and σ_x the standard deviation (SD) of the sample values. Parameter k is higher for more peaked signals.

The parameter cr was calculated as the width/height of the CR expansion. The width of the CR expansion was defined at the level of 50 crossings/second and the height as the maximum value of the CR expansion. Parameter cr is lower for more peaked signals.

3.2.2. EMG parameters of nonlinear dynamics

In [28, 29], we used parameters of nonlinear dynamics (correlation dimension, recurrence rate and cross-recurrence rate) for analyzing the EMG signal complexity and recurring EMG patterns. In nonlinear dynamics, the original time series (EMG signal) x is used to form embedding vectors u_i

$$u_i = [x_i \; x_{i+\lambda} \; x_{i+2\lambda} \; \cdots \; x_{i+(m-1)\lambda}], \tag{5}$$

where λ is the delay parameter and m the embedding dimension [45]. The number of different embedding vectors is $N_m = N_e - (m-1)\lambda$ for each epoch (length N_e) of the time series x.

The correlation dimension [16] describes the complexity of the time series and it can be calculated from the embedding vectors as follows. First, the Euclidean distances between each pair of embedding vectors u_i and u_j in (5) are quantified as

$$d_e(u_i, u_j) = \sqrt{\sum_{k=0}^{m-1} |x_{i+k\lambda} - x_{j+k\lambda}|^2}. \tag{6}$$

The correlation sum is then calculated as

$$C^m(r) = \frac{1}{N_m^2} \sum_{i,j=1}^{N_m} \Theta(r - d_e(u_i, u_j)) \tag{7}$$

$$\Theta(s) = \begin{cases} 0, & s < 0 \\ 1, & s \geq 0, \end{cases}$$

where r is the threshold distance. The correlation dimension is formally defined as

$$D_2(m) = \lim_{r \to 0} \lim_{N_m \to \infty} \frac{\log C^m(r)}{\log r}. \tag{8}$$

Practically, D_2 is calculated as the slope of the regression curve in the log-log-representation.

Recurrence rate [53] measures the percentage of recurring patterns in the EMG signal. It can be calculated from the embedding vector distances in (6) as a percentage of distances that are below of the threshold distance r. The binary image, that contains a value 1 in the cells (i, j) where $d_e(u_i, u_j) < r$, is called the recurrence plot. The recurrence plots of one healthy subject and one PD patient are illustrated in Figure 4. One can observe that the recurrence plot of the patient contains more cells with the value 1 (white cells) than the recurrence plot of the healthy subject. It means that the EMG signal of the patient contains more recurring patterns than the EMG signal of the healthy subject. In the cross-recurrence rate, the embedding vectors in (5) are formed for two time series and the Euclidean distances in (6) are evaluated between the embedding vectors of the two different time series.

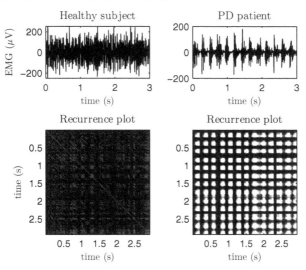

Figure 4. EMG signals and recurrence plots of one healthy subject and one PD patient.

3.2.3. Spectral-based parameters

In spectral analysis, the aim is to present the signal in the frequency-domain by estimating its power spectral density (PSD). The PSD estimation can be based on a Fourier transform or wavelet transform or on parametric modeling. In [28, 29], the Fourier- and wavelet-based approaches were used for analyzing the EMG and acceleration signals of PD patients and healthy subjects.

The coherence was used in [28] for quantifying similarities in the power spectra of the EMG and acceleration signals. It was calculated from the PSDs of the EMG and acceleration signals ($P_x(f)$ and $P_y(f)$) and from the cross-spectral density $P_{xy}(f)$, which were estimated by using the Welch's averaged periodogram method [54]. The magnitude-squared coherence is defined as

$$C_{xy}(f) = \frac{|P_{xy}(f)|^2}{P_x(f)P_y(f)} \tag{9}$$

and it gives values between 0 and 1. Variable Coh was calculated as the area of the coherence spectrum above a threshold value in the frequency range 0–50 Hz. The magnitude-squared coherence estimates of one healthy subject and one PD patient are presented in Figure 5. One can observe that the area of the coherence spectrum is larger for the PD patient than for the healthy subject.

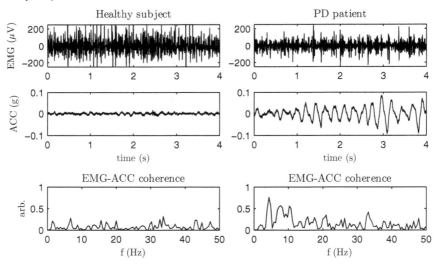

Figure 5. EMG and acceleration signals and magnitude-squared coherence estimates of one healthy subject and one PD patient.

While in Fourier approach the basis functions in the spectral decomposition are global functions, in wavelet approach [1] the functions are local. Therefore, the wavelet-based methods can be more effective than the Fourier-based method in detecting time varying features in the spectrum [10]. The basic idea in the wavelet transform is to decompose the signal into a set of basis functions, which are obtained by scaling and shifting the wavelet function $\psi(t)$. In continuous form, the wavelet transform of the signal $x(t)$ is defined as

$$W_x(a,b) = \frac{1}{\sqrt{a}} \int_{-\infty}^{\infty} x(t)\psi^* \left(\frac{t-b}{a} \right) dt, \tag{10}$$

where a is the scale, b is the shift, and $(\cdot)^*$ denotes the complex conjugate operator. Different kinds of wavelet functions have been defined for analysis. For discrete signals one must use discrete wavelets. The magnitude-squared wavelet transform is called the scalogram

$$P_x^W(a,b) = |W_x(a,b)W_x^*(a,b)|. \tag{11}$$

If the wavelet transforms of two signals x and y are denoted with $W_x(a,b)$ and $W_y(a,b)$, the wavelet cross-scalogram is defined as

$$P_{xy}^W(a,b) = |W_x(a,b)W_y^*(a,b)|. \tag{12}$$

In [29], the discrete Morlet wavelet was used for analysis as in many other EMG studies [10, 20, 40]. The scalograms (11) were calculated from the EMG signals of both sides of the body and the cross-scalogram (12) between the right and left side signals. The scalograms and cross-scalograms were scaled to present the percentage of energy for each wavelet coefficient as a function of time. The wavelet parameter $W_{\max}$ was calculated as the maximum energy of all wavelet coefficients from both the scalograms and the cross-scalograms as a function of time. The wavelet cross-scalograms and parameters $W_{\max,rl}$ are presented for one healthy subject and one PD patient in Figure 6. One can observe that in the wavelet cross-scalogram of the patient the energy is more spread into different wavelet coefficients than in the cross-scalogram of the healthy subject. Parameter $W_{\max,rl}$ is lower for the patient.

3.2.4. Acceleration signal features

Sample entropy is a parameter of nonlinear dynamics and it can be used for quantifying the regularity of acceleration signals in PD when compared to the healthy subjects. It was calculated in [28, 29] from the embedding vectors in (5) as described in [27]. In [29], the power of the acceleration signal was extracted from the dynamic acceleration recordings for quantifying kinetic tremor and rigidity during movement.

3.3. Cluster analysis of subjects

The aim in [28, 29] was to develop a method for discriminating between PD patients and healthy subjects on the basis of EMG and accelerations signal features. In total, the data from 42 PD patients and 59 healthy subjects were analyzed in [28] and the data from 49 PD patients and 59 healthy subjects were analyzed in [29].

In [28, 29], there were many parameters that could capture essential information in the measured signals. These original signal features p_j $(j = 1, 2, ..., N_p)$ (detailed in Table 1) were used to form feature vectors $z_j \in \mathbb{R}^{N_p}$ for each subject.

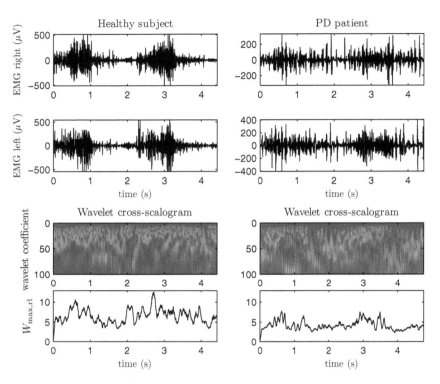

Figure 6. Right and left side EMG signals of one healthy subject and one PD patient. Wavelet cross-scalograms and $W_{max,rl}$ parameters for the healthy subject and the PD patient.

$$z_j = [p_1 \ p_2 \ldots p_{N_p}]^T \tag{13}$$

The PC-based approach [19] was used in both studies for reducing the number signal features and for transforming the original possibly correlated parameters into uncorrelated parameters.

In [28], one feature vector was formed for each healthy subject, for each patient with medication on (MED on) and for 13 patients also with medication off (MED off, no medication 24 hours before the measurement) by using the twelve EMG and acceleration parameters (six parameters from each body side) that are detailed in Table 1. The original signal parameters were normalized (to zero mean and unit SD of all subjects) before applying the PC approach. The PC approach was applied once as described in section 2.2. In [29], two feature vectors were formed for each patient and for each healthy subject of the ten EMG and acceleration parameters that are detailed in Table 1. One of the feature vectors was formed by using the mean parameter values during flexion and the other by using the mean parameter values during extension. The signal variables were normalized and the PC approach was applied separately for the flexion and extension phases of the movement as described in section 2.2.

Cluster analysis was used in [28, 29] for grouping subjects with similar EMG and acceleration signal features into groups. This could be done by clustering the model weights (PCs) in the sum (1). An iterative k-means algorithm [47] was used for clustering the feature vectors of subjects in a two-dimensional feature space. In k-means algorithm, the only parameter given to the algorithm is the number of clusters. The algorithm begins by choosing initial estimates for each cluster center point. In each iteration step, it is determined to which cluster the feature vectors belong. The feature vector belongs to that cluster for which the squared Euclidean distance between the vector and the cluster center point in the two-dimensional feature space is minimized. The cluster center points are updated to be the mean of the feature vectors in each cluster in the two-dimensional feature space. The iteration continues until the sum of vector-to-center point distances summed over all clusters is minimized.

The validation of the clustering results was performed by using the leave-one-out method. In the method, the eigenvectors and PCs are solved for each combination of $M - 1$ feature vectors, where M means the total number of feature vectors. That is, one feature vector is left out of the group each time the eigenvectors and PCs are computed. The clustering is then performed for each combination of $M - 1$ feature vectors, and in each case, it is tested to which cluster the feature vector that was left out belongs. In [28, 29], the correct ratings of clustering were defined as the percentage (mean±SD values) of healthy subjects that belong to the healthy subject cluster and the percentage of patients that belong to the patient clusters.

3.4. Discrimination results

In [28], twelve features were extracted from the isometric EMG and acceleration signals of 59 healthy subjects and 42 PD patients. The normalized signal features (mean±SD values) for the healthy subject group and for the PD patient group are presented in Figure 7. The results show that the parameters SampEn, cr and D_2 seem to be lower and the parameters k, Coh and %REC higher for the patients than for the healthy subjects. That is, the EMGs of the patients tend to be less complex and contain more recurring patterns than the EMGs of the healthy subjects. The acceleration signals of the patients tend to be more regular and more coherent with the EMGs than the acceleration signals of the healthy subjects.

The cluster analysis of subjects was performed in a two-dimensional feature space, that was spanned by the PC sum $\theta_j(2) + \theta_j(5)$ and the first PC $\theta_j(1)$ by using the k-means algorithm. This PC sum was used, because it works better in discrimination than the single PCs. The results in Figure 7 show that 90 % of the healthy subjects belong to the cluster O_1 and 76 % of the patients in two other clusters O_2 and O_3. Seven patients with severe motor symptoms are distinguished in O_3. The ten patients in the healthy subject cluster O_1 have only little or no tremor at all in their hands. The validation by using the leave-one-out method resulted in correct discrimination rates of 90 ± 1 % for the healthy subjects and 74 ± 6 % for the patients.

In [29], ten features were extracted from the EMG and acceleration signals of 59 healthy subjects and 49 PD patients and used to form feature vectors for subjects. The normalized signal features (mean±SD values) for the healthy subject group and for the PD patient group

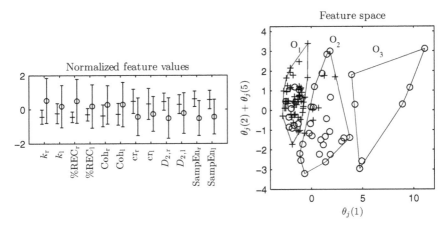

Figure 7. Mean ± SD values of normalized signal features for the patient group (∘) and for the healthy subject group (+) (left). The cluster analysis of 42 PD patients (∘) and 59 healthy subjects (+) in the feature space $(\theta_j(2)+\theta_j(5)$ with respect to $\theta_j(1))$. The three clusters O_1, O_2 and O_3.

in flexion and in extension are presented in Figure 8. The results show that parameters %REC and P_{acc} tend to be higher and parameters SampEn and W_{max} lower for patients than for healthy subjects both in flexion and in extension. That is, the EMGs of the patients tend to contain more recurring patterns than the EMGs of the healthy subjects and the EMG wavelet power tends to be more spread for patients. The acceleration signals of the patients tend to be of higher amplitude and more regular than the acceleration signals of the healthy subjects.

The cluster analysis of subjects was performed in a two-dimensional feature space that was spanned by the second PC and the first PC by using the k-means algorithm. The results are presented in Figure 8. According to the results, the method can discriminate 80 ± 1 % of the patient extension movements from 87 ± 1 % of the extension movements of healthy subjects, and 73 ± 1 % of the patient flexion movements from 82 ± 1 % of the flexion movements of healthy subjects. The leave-one-out method was used for validation. The patients, that could not be discriminated from the healthy subjects, had mild motor symptoms of PD.

4. PC-based approaches for quantifying effects of treatment

In addition to the discrimination analysis between subjects, the principal component -based approach can be used for quantifying the effects of treatment. In [30, 31], we aimed to develop objective methods for quantifying effects of PD treatment (DBS and medication) on the basis of surface EMG and acceleration measurements and analysis.

4.1. EMG and acceleration measurements for quantifying effects of treatment

In [30], the PC-based approach was used for quantifying the effects of DBS treatment on the basis of a set of EMG and acceleration signal features. In total, the measurement data from 13 PD patients with DBS and 13 healthy subjects were analyzed. Measurements were performed

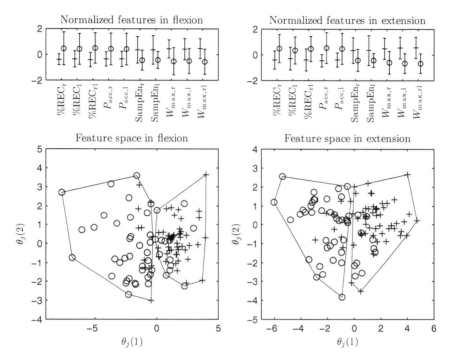

Figure 8. Mean ± SD values of normalized signal features for the patient group (○) and for the healthy subject group (+) in flexion and in extension (top). The cluster analysis of 49 PD patients (○) and 59 healthy subjects (+) in the feature space ($\theta_j(2)$ with respect to $\theta_j(1)$).

during the isometric contraction of BB muscles (see section 3.1) and they were performed once for the healthy subjects and twice for the patients: with DBS on (stimulator was turned on) and with DBS off (stimulator was turned off). Ninth order Butterworth low-pass filter with 110 Hz cutoff was used for removing the DBS artifact from the EMG signals. The low-pass filtering was performed similarly for all subjects (patients and healthy subjects). The UPDRS -motor examination was performed for each patient with DBS on and with DBS off. The measured signals of one PD patient with DBS on and off are presented in Figure 9. One can observe that the EMG signal of the patient contains recurring EMG bursts and the acceleration signal high-amplitude tremor with DBS off but not with DBS on.

In [31], the PC-based approach was used for quantifying the effects of anti-parkinsonian medication on the basis of a set of EMG and acceleration signal features. In total, the measurement data from nine PD patients were analyzed. The subjects were measured in four different medication conditions: off-medication, and two and three and four hours after taking the medication. The isometric task (described in section 3.1) was analyzed. The UPDRS -motor examination was performed for each patient in each medication condition. The EMG and acceleration signals of one PD patient in each medication condition are presented in Figure

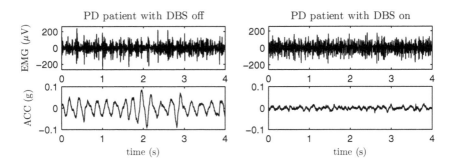

Figure 9. The EMG and acceleration signals of one PD patient with DBS on and with DBS off.

10. It is observed that the number of recurring EMG bursts and the amplitude of tremor decrease with medication and start to increase three hours after taking the medication.

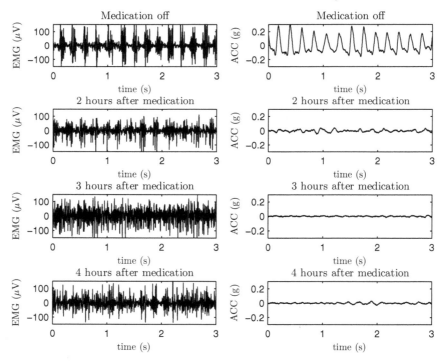

Figure 10. The EMG and acceleration signals of one PD patient in four medication conditions: with medication off, and two and three and four hours after taking the medication.

4.2. EMG and acceleration signal features for characterizing effects of treatment

Several EMG and acceleration signal features were observed to be effective in characterizing the effects of treatment on PD patients in [30, 31]. These features are detailed in Table 2.

Treatment	Signal features	Notations
DBS	correlation dimension of EMG	$D_{2,r}$ and $D_{2,l}$
	recurrence rate of EMG	%REC$_r$ and %REC$_l$
	root mean square amplitude of ACC	RMS$_r$ and RMS$_l$
	sample entropy of ACC	SampEn$_r$ and SampEn$_l$
	coherence between EMG and ACC	Coh$_r$ and Coh$_l$
Medication	sample kurtosis of EMG	k_r and k_l
	recurrence rate of EMG	%REC$_r$ and %REC$_l$
	root mean square amplitude of ACC	RMS$_r$ and RMS$_l$
	sample entropy of ACC	SampEn$_r$ and SampEn$_l$

Table 2. PD characteristic signal features for quantifying effects of treatment. The subscripts r and l in the notations stand for the side of the body.

The parameters were calculated as described in section 3.2. The root mean square amplitude of acceleration was calculated for quantifying tremor amplitude.

4.3. Principal components in quantifying the effects of treatment

In [30], the ten signal features (five features from each body side) in Table 2 were normalized (to zero mean and unit SD of healthy subjects) and used to form feature vectors for subjects. One feature vector was formed for each healthy subject and two feature vectors for each patient: one with DBS on and one with DBS off. The PC approach (see section 2.2) was applied once. The eigenvectors were solved by using the feature vectors of healthy subjects. In this way, the healthy subject group formed the normal group for later comparison.

In [31], the eight signal parameters in Table 2 were normalized (to zero mean and unit SD of all patients) and used to form feature vectors for PD patients. Four feature vectors were formed for each patient (one feature vector in each medication condition). The PC approach (see section 2.2) was applied once.

4.4. Results

In [30], the group mean values of the parameters D_2 and SampEn increased and the group mean values of the parameters %REC, RMS and Coh decreased with DBS for the patient group. However, the SDs of the parameters were very high for the patient group because of its heterogeneity. Therefore, the patient measurements were studied individually. The first and the third PCs worked best in characterizing effects of DBS and differences between patients and healthy subjects. According to the results in Figure 11, 12 out of 13 patients are closer to the center point of healthy subjects with DBS on than with DBS off in the two-dimensional feature space ($\theta_3(j)$ with respect to $\theta_1(j)$). That is, the EMG and acceleration signals of PD patients are more similar with the signals of the healthy subjects with DBS on than with DBS off. The distances of the patients from the center of healthy subjects and the clinical UPDRS -motor scores are highly individual (see Table 3). It was observed in a more detailed analysis that the method is most sensitive to PD with associated tremor. In Figure 11, one patient is farther from the healthy subjects with DBS on than with DBS off. This patient has higher tremor (acceleration signal) amplitude and regularity and less complex EMG recordings (higher %REC and lower D_2) with DBS on than with DBS off. For that patient, the measurement results contradict the subjective clinical scores.

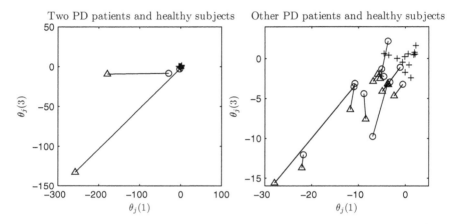

Figure 11. The third PCs $\theta_j(3)$ with respect to the first PCs $\theta_j(1)$ of 13 healthy subjects (+) and 13 PD patients with DBS on (○) and off (△). The patients are divided into two figures, but the healthy subjects are the same in both figures. The DBS on- and off-states of each patient are connected with a line.

In [31], the first PC worked best in characterizing the effects of medication. The first PCs and the total UPDRS -motor scores in each medication condition for each patient are presented in Figure 12. One can observe that the total UPDRS -motor scores decrease (motor symptoms are relieved) with medication for all patients. Correspondingly the first PCs decrease with medication for eight out of nine patients. By examining the first eigenvector in Figure 12 one can realize that the reduction in the first PC indicates reduction in the parameters k (less spiky EMG), %REC (less recurring patterns) and RMS (lower tremor amplitude), and increase in the parameter SampEn (more complex tremor). The severity of motor symptoms (UPDRS -motor score) starts to increase 2–3 hours after medication for all patients, which indicates that the efficacy of medication starts to weaken 2–3 hours after medication. Correspondingly, the first PCs start to increase 2–3 hours after medication for seven out of nine patients. The UPDRS -motor scores and the first PCs do not start to increase at the same time for all patients, which indicates that these scores do not measure exactly the same thing.

5. Discussion

There is a need for finding objective methods for Parkinson's disease for improving the diagnostic accuracy, for enabling earlier diagnosis, and for quantifying the disease progression and the efficacy of treatment [2, 11, 24]. Surface EMG and the kinematic measurements may be potentially useful methods for quantifying the motor impairment in PD and the effects of

Patient no.	UPDRS off	UPDRS on	Distance off	Distance on
1	56	43	26	25
2	64	48	32	12
3	59	40	7	5
4	34	14	180	30
5	71	42	289	4
6	38	31	5	12
7	47	28	6	2
8	57	33	6	4
9	43	34	13	11
10	43	24	11	10
11	44	30	6	5
12	62	38	5	4
13	43	30	5	3

Table 3. Total UPDRS -motor scores and the distances from the center of healthy subjects with DBS on and off.

treatment. However, the EMG signals of PD patients are characterized by spikes and bursts that are not effectively captured with conventional amplitude- and spectral-based parameters of EMG. Therefore, more novel methods of EMG analysis are needed for PD.

5.1. Discrimination between patients and healthy subjects

We have developed methods for discriminating between PD patients and healthy subjects on the basis of surface EMG and kinematic measurements and analysis in [28, 29, 32]. One developed approach was based on analyzing the surface EMG signal morphology [32]. One approach was based on analyzing isometric [28] and one approach on analyzing dynamic muscle contractions [29]. Principal components were used in each approach for discrimination between subjects. All methods were tested with the measured data. The obtained discrimination rates were 72 % for patients and 86 % for healthy subjects on the basis of surface EMG signal morphology, 76 % for patients and 90 % for healthy subjects on the basis of isometric EMG and acceleration recordings, 73 % for patients and 82 % for healthy subjects on the basis of elbow flexion movements, and 80 % for patients and 87 % for healthy subjects on the basis of elbow extension movements. These percentages predict the sensitivities and specificities of the methods in the subject groups that were studied.

The best discrimination rates between patients and healthy subjects were obtained by analyzing the EMG and acceleration signals measured during the isometric contraction and elbow extension movements [28, 29]. In fact, it has been observed previously, that the elbow extension movements are more impaired than the flexion movements of PD patients [33]. The isometric approach was most sensitive to patients with associated tremor [28] and the dynamic approach to patients with various motor symptoms (rigidity, bradykinesia and tremor) and

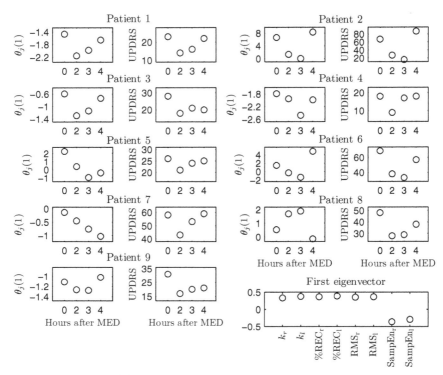

Figure 12. The first PCs ($\theta_j(1)$) and UPDRS -motor scores of nine PD patients with medication off, and two and three and hour hours after taking the medication. The first eigenvector (bottom right).

especially to patients with problems in performing movement tasks [29]. Therefore, the analysis of both kind of muscle contractions is essential when quantifying motor impairment in PD.

5.2. Quantification of the effects of treatment

In studies [30, 31], we developed methods for quantifying the effects of treatment in PD on the basis of surface EMG and kinematic measurements and analysis. The results of the study [30] show that the measured EMG and acceleration signals of 12 out of 13 PD patients were more similar with the signals of the healthy subjects with DBS on than with DBS off. This result indicates that it is possible to detect DBS-induced improvements in the neuromuscular and motor function of PD patients by using the developed analysis approach.

In [31], the EMG signals of eight out of nine PD patients changed into less spiky and the acceleration recordings into more complex after taking the medication. A reverse phenomenon in the signal characteristics was observed 3–4 hours after taking the medication for seven out of nine patients. This result indicates that it is possible to detect medication-induced changes in the neuromuscular and motor function of PD patients by using the developed methods.

5.3. Methods of signal analysis

We extracted a large number of features from the EMG and acceleration signals of PD patients and healthy subjects in [28–32] and chose the most effective features for characterizing PD and the effects of treatment into the feature vectors for deeper analysis. The chosen EMG features were not conventional EMG parameters but they were based on nonlinear dynamics, signal morphology, wavelets and EMG-acceleration coherence. Previously, there have been only one [14] or few other studies, in which a method of nonlinear dynamics has been used for studying EMGs of PD patients. Our studies [30, 31] are the only studies that have analyzed the effects of PD treatment (DBS and medication) by using methods of nonlinear dynamics for EMG.

All of the studies [28–32] were based on an innovative way of combining the PC-based approach with the selection of feature vectors instead of analyzing the statistics of single signal parameters. The PC-based approach provided a better discrimination between the subjects by capturing essential information in the combination of variables. With the PC-based approach, it was possible to examine the effects of treatment in a feature space on an individual level.

Few things about signal quality and electrode placement should be kept in mind when analyzing the EMG signals with the proposed analysis methods. First, the EMG signal amplitude is relatively low and the signal is sensitive to noise that is coming from other electrical sources. This noise may affect the calculated signal parameters. Therefore, the noise should be eliminated already during the measurements whenever it is possible. Another thing is that sometimes a large MU is firing constantly and dominantly in the proximity of the recording electrode causing recurring impulse-like patterns into the EMG signal. In that case, a better placement of recording electrodes would be advisable.

In PD patients with DBS, the stimulator causes artifacts into the EMG signal. The DBS artifact and its filtering may affect the calculated signal parameters. Previously, the DBS artifact has been removed from the EMG signal by low-pass filtering the rectified signal with a low (20–60 Hz) cut-off frequency [21, 41, 42, 51, 52]. In our study [30], we low-pass filtered the EMG signal with the 110 Hz cut-off frequency. Our aim was to remove the DBS artifact from the EMG as effectively as possible without removing important information and to perform the filtering in the same way for all subjects in order to get comparable results.

5.4. Conclusions

In this chapter, we presented several approaches for feature extraction from surface EMG and acceleration signals and for discrimination between PD patients and healthy subjects on the basis of the extracted signal features. The presented discrimination approaches were developed in our studies [28, 29, 32]. By using the developed approaches, we could discriminate 72-80 % of PD patients from 82-90 % of healthy subjects depending on the analyzed signal features and the muscle contraction type. These percentages can be regarded as promising because it is known that the PD diagnostics can be difficult. Clinicopathological studies from the UK and Canada have shown that the disease is diagnosed incorrectly in about 25 % of cases [48]. On the basis of our discrimination results, further research and clinical studies are suggested for evaluating the sensitivity of the developed approaches in patients with different types of PD and in patients with early stages of PD. In addition, the ability of EMG and acceleration signal features in discriminating between PD patients and other patients with similar symptoms should be studied.

In this chapter, we presented two approaches for quantifying the effects of PD treatment (medication and DBS) on the basis of the extracted EMG and acceleration signal features. The presented approaches were developed in our studies [30, 31]. By using the developed approaches, we could detect DBS- and medication-induced improvements in the neuromuscular and motor function of PD patients. This result is encouraging because the widely used method for evaluating the efficacy of PD treatment is subjective. However, the sensitivity of the developed approaches should be quantified with a larger number of PD patients.

The need for finding objective methods for PD diagnosis and for quantifying the disease progression and the efficacy of treatment is well known [2, 11, 24]. We hope that our results [28–32] can help in creating a practical method for quantifying motor impairment in PD and the effects of treatment on individual PD patients. However, in order to be more sensitive than the traditional methods, it is probable that a combination of several objective methods will be needed for PD.

5.5. Future directions

There is currently a lot of effort for determining objective methods and characteristics for PD [2, 11, 24]. One important goal of current research is to determine criteria for the pre-motor and pre-clinical phases of PD [39]. In surface EMG studies, the sensitivity of surface EMG signal features in detecting PD patients before the actual diagnosis of PD should be studied. It will be important to analyze differences in the signal characteristics between PD patients and other patients with similar symptoms. These other similar diseases form currently a significant reason for the wrong diagnosis of PD [17]. It has been observed that surface EMG and kinematic measurements can provide information about the effects of PD treatments (medication and DBS). The ability of these measurements in helping the optimal adjustment of these treatments should be evaluated.

Acknowledgments

This work was supported by the Academy of Finland under Project 252748.

Author details

Rissanen Saara M., Tarvainen Mika P. and Karjalainen Pasi A.
Department of Applied Physics, University of Eastern Finland, Kuopio, Finland

Kankaanpää Markku
Department of Physical and Rehabilitation Medicine, Tampere University Hospital, Tampere, Finland

6. References

[1] Akay, M. [1998]. *Time frequency and wavelets in biomedical signal processing*, IEEE Press
series in biomedical engineering, IEEE Press, New York.

[2] Antoniades, C. & Barker, R. [2008]. The search for biomarkers in Parkinson's disease: a
critical review, *Expert Rev. Neurother.* 8(12): 1841–1852.

[3] Bastian, A., Kelly, V., Revilla, F., Perlmutter, J. & Mink, J. [2003]. Different effects of
unilateral versus bilateral subthalamic nucleus stimulation on walking and reaching in
Parkinson's disease, *Mov. Disord.* 18(9): 1000–1007.

[4] Blahak, C., Wöhrle, J., Capelle, H.-H., Bäzner, H., Grips, E., Weigel, R., Hennerici, M. &
Krauss, J. [2007]. Tremor reduction by subthalamic nucleus stimulation and medication
in advanced Parkinson's disease, *J. Neurol.* 254(2): 169–178.

[5] Carpinella, I., Crenna, P., Calabrese, E., Rabuffetti, M., Mazzoleni, P., Nemni, R. &
Ferrarin, M. [2007]. Locomotor function in the early stage of Parkinson's disease, *IEEE
Trans. Neural. Syst. Rehabil. Eng.* 15(4): 543–551.

[6] Carpinella, I., Crenna, P., Marzegan, A., Rabuffetti, M., Rizzone, M., Lopiano, L. &
Ferrarin [2007]. Effect of l-dopa and subthalamic nucleus stimulation on arm and
leg swing during gait in Parkinson's disease, *Conf. Proc. IEEE Eng. Med. Biol. Soc.*,
pp. 6665–6668.

[7] Chastan, N., Westby, G., Yelnik, J., Bardinet, E., Do, M., Agid, Y. & Welter, M. [2009].
Effects of nigral stimulation on locomotion and postural stability in patients with
Parkinson's disease, *Brain* 132(1): 172–184.

[8] Dafotakis, M., Fink, G., Allert, N. & Nowak, D. [2008]. The impact of subthalamic
deep brain stimulation on bradykinesia of proximal and distal upper limb muscles in
Parkinson's disease, *J. Neurol.* 255(3): 429–437.

[9] de Lau, L. & Breteler, M. [2006]. Epidemiology of Parkinson's disease, *Lancet Neurol.*
5(6): 525–535.

[10] de Michele, G., Sello, S., Carboncini, M., Rossi, B. & Strambi, S.-K. [2003].
Cross-correlation time-frequency analysis for multiple EMG signals in Parkinson's
disease: a wavelet approach, *Med. Eng. Phys.* 25(5): 361–369.

[11] Dorsey, E., Holloway, R. & Ravina, B. [2008]. Status of biological markers, *in* S. Factor &
W. Weiner (eds), *Parkinson's disease: diagnosis and clinical management (2nd Edition)*, Demos
Medical Publishing, Inc., New York, chapter 24, pp. 277–284.

[12] Fahn, S. & Elton, R. [1987]. The Unified Parkinson's disease rating scale, *in* S. Fahn,
C. Marsden, D. Calne & M. Goldstein (eds), *Recent developments in Parkinson's disease*,
Macmillan Healthcare Information, Florham Park, N.J., pp. 153–63.

[13] Farley, B., Sherman, S. & Koshland, G. [2004]. Shoulder muscle activity in Parkinson's
disease during multijoint arm movements across a range of speeds, *Exp. Brain Res.*
154(2): 160–175.

[14] Fattorini, L., Felici, F., Filligoi, G., Traballesi, M. & Farina, D. [2005]. Influence of high
motor unit synchronization levels on non-linear and spectral variables of the surface
EMG, *J. Neurosci. Methods* 143(2): 133–139.

[15] Gancher, S. [2008]. Clinical rating scales, *in* S. Factor & W. Weiner (eds), *Parkinson's
disease: diagnosis and clinical management (2nd Edition)*, Demos Medical Publishing, Inc.,
New York, chapter 14, pp. 135–143.

[16] Grassberger, P. & Procaccia, I. [1983]. Characterization of strange attractors, *Phys. Rev. Lett.* 50(5): 346–349.

[17] Grosset, D., Grosset, K., Okun, M. & Fernandez, H. [2009]. *Parkinson's disease - Clinician's desk reference*, Manson Publishing Ltd., London.

[18] Jankovic, J. [2008]. Parkinson's disease: clinical features and diagnosis, *J. Neurol. Neurosurg. Psychiatry* 79(4): 368–376.

[19] Jolliffe, I. [2002]. *Principal Component Analysis*, Springer-Verlag, New York.

[20] Karlsson, S., Yu, J. & Akay, M. [2000]. Time-frequency analysis of myoelectric signals during dynamic contractions: A comparative study, *IEEE Trans. Biomed. Eng.* 47(2): 228–238.

[21] Levin, J., Krafczyk, S., Valkovič, P., Eggert, T., Claassen, J. & Bötzel, K. [2009]. Objective measurement of muscle rigidity in parkinsonian patients treated with subthalamic stimulation, *Mov. Disord.* 24(1): 57–63.

[22] Marek, K., Jennings, D., Tamagnan, G. & Seibyl, J. [2008]. Biomarkers for Parkinson's disease: tools to assess Parkinson's disease onset and progression, *Ann. Neurol.* 64 (suppl. 2): S111–S121.

[23] Meigal, A., Rissanen, S., Tarvainen, M., Karjalainen, P., Iudina-Vassel, I., Airaksinen, O. & Kankaanpää, M. [2009]. Novel parameters of surface EMG in patients with Parkinson's disease and healthy young and old controls, *J. Electromyogr. Kinesiol.* 19(3): e206–e213.

[24] Morgan, J., Mehta, S. & Sethi, K. [2010]. Biomarkers in Parkinson's disease, *Curr. Neurol. Neurosci. Rep.* 10(6): 423–430.

[25] Park, H., Kim, J., Paek, S., Jeon, B., Lee, J. & Chung, C. [2009]. Cortico-muscular coherence increases with tremor improvement after deep brain stimulation in Parkinson's disease, *Neuroreport* 20(16): 1444–1449.

[26] Pfann, K., Buchman, A., Comella, C. & Corcos, D. [2001]. Control of movement distance in Parkinson's disease, *Mov. Disord.* 16(6): 1048–1065.

[27] Richman, J. & Moorman, J. [2000]. Physiological time-series analysis using approximate entropy and sample entropy, *Am. J. Physiol. Heart Circ. Physiol.* 278(6): H2039–H2049.

[28] Rissanen, S., Kankaanpää, M., Meigal, A., Tarvainen, M., Nuutinen, J., Tarkka, I., Airaksinen, O. & Karjalainen, P. [2008]. Surface EMG and acceleration signals in Parkinson's disease: feature extraction and cluster analysis, *Med. Biol. Eng. Comput.* 46(9): 849–858.

[29] Rissanen, S., Kankaanpää, M., Tarvainen, M., Meigal, A., Nuutinen, J., Tarkka, I., Airaksinen, O. & Karjalainen, P. [2009]. Analysis of dynamic voluntary muscle contractions in Parkinson's disease, *IEEE Trans. Biomed. Eng.* 56(9): 2280–2288.

[30] Rissanen, S., Kankaanpää, M., Tarvainen, M., Novak, V., Novak, P., Hu, K., Manor, B., Airaksinen, O. & Karjalainen, P. [2011]. Analysis of EMG and acceleration signals for quantifying the effects of deep brain stimulation in Parkinson's disease, *IEEE Trans. Biomed. Eng.* 58(9): 2545–2553.

[31] Rissanen, S., Kankaanpää, M., Tarvainen, M., Nuutinen, J., Airaksinen, O. & Karjalainen, P. [2011]. EMG and acceleration signal analysis for quantifying the effects of medication in Parkinson's disease, *Conf. Proc. IEEE Eng. Med. Biol. Soc.*, pp. 7496–7499.

[32] Rissanen, S., Kankaanpää, M., Tarvainen, M., Nuutinen, J., Tarkka, I., Airaksinen, O. & Karjalainen, P. [2007]. Analysis of surface EMG signal morphology in Parkinson's disease, *Physiol. Meas.* 28(12): 1507–1521.

[33] Robichaud, J., Pfann, K., Comella, C., Brandabur, M. & Corcos, D. [2004]. Greater impairment of extension movements as compared to flexion movements in Parkinson's disease, *Exp. Brain Res.* 156(2): 240–254.

[34] Robichaud, J., Pfann, K., Comella, C. & Corcos, D. [2002]. Effect of medication on EMG patterns in individuals with Parkinson's disease, *Mov. Disord.* 17(5): 950–960.

[35] Robichaud, J., Pfann, K., Leurgans, S., Vaillancourt, D., Comella, C. & Corcos, D. [2009]. Variability of EMG patterns: a potential neurophysiological marker of Parkinson's disease, *Clin. Neurophysiol.* 120(2): 390–397.

[36] Roiz, R., Cacho, E., Pazinatto, M., Reis, J., Cliquet, A. & Barasnevicius-Quagliato, E. [2010]. Gait analysis comparing Parkinson's disease with healthy elderly subjects., *Arq. Neuropsiquiatr.* 68(1): 81–86.

[37] Salenius, S., Avikainen, S., Kaakkola, S., Hari, R. & Brown, P. [2002]. Defective cortical drive to muscle in Parkinson's disease and its improvement with levodopa, *Brain* 125(3): 491–500.

[38] Savica, R., Rocca, W. & Ahlskog, J. [2010]. When does Parkinson disease start?, *Arch. Neurol.* 67(7): 798–801.

[39] Stern, M., Lang, A. & Poewe, W. [2012]. Toward a redefinition of Parkinson's disease?, *Mov. Disord.* 27(1): 54–60.

[40] Strambi, S., Rossi, B., de Michele, G. & Sello, S. [2004]. Effect of medication in Parkinson's disease: a wavelet analysis of EMG signals, *Med. Eng. Phys.* 26(4): 279–290.

[41] Sturman, M., Vaillancourt, D., Metman, L., Bakay, R. & Corcos, D. [2004]. Effects of subthalamic nucleus stimulation and medication on resting and postural tremor in Parkinson's disease, *Brain* 127(9): 2131–2143.

[42] Sturman, M., Vaillancourt, D., Metman, L., Sierens, D., Bakay, R. & Corcos, D. [2007]. Deep brain stimulation and medication for parkinsonian tremor during secondary tasks, *Mov. Disord.* 22(8): 1157–1163.

[43] Svehlík, M., Zwick, E., Steinwender, G., Linhart, W., Schwingenschuh, P., Katschnig, P., Ott, E. & Enzinger, C. [2009]. Gait analysis in patients with Parkinson's disease off dopaminergic therapy, *Arch. Phys. Med. Rehabil.* 90(11): 1880–1886.

[44] Tabbal, S., Ushe, M., Mink, J., Revilla, F., Wernle, A., Hong, M., Karimi, M. & Perlmutter, J. [2008]. Unilateral subthalamic nucleus stimulation has a measurable ipsilateral effect on rigidity and bradykinesia in Parkinson disease, *Exp. Neurol.* 211(1): 234–242.

[45] Takens, F. [1981]. Detecting strange attractors in turbulence, *in* D. Rand & L.-S. Young (eds), *Dynamical Systems and Turbulence, Warwick 1980*, Vol. 898 of *Lecture Notes in Mathematics*, Springer Berlin / Heidelberg, pp. 366–381.

[46] Tarvainen, M., Ranta-aho, P. & Karjalainen, P. [2002]. An advanced detrending method with application to HRV analysis, *IEEE Trans. Biomed. Eng.* 49(2): 172–175.

[47] Theodoridis, S. & Koutroumbas, K. [2006]. *Pattern recognition*, Elsevier/Academic Press, USA.

[48] Tolosa, E., Wenning, G. & Poewe, W. [2006]. The diagnosis of Parkinson's disease, *Lancet Neurol.* 5(1): 75–86.

[49] Tucha, O., Mecklinger, L., Thome, J., Reiter, A., Alders, G., Sartor, H., Naumann, M. & Lange, K. [2006]. Kinematic analysis of dopaminergic effects on skilled handwriting movements in Parkinson's disease, *J. Neural. Transm.* 113(5): 609–623.

[50] Vaillancourt, D. & Newell, K. [2000]. The dynamics of resting and postural tremor in Parkinson's disease, *Clin. Neurophysiol.* 111(11): 2046–2056.

[51] Vaillancourt, D., Prodoehl, J., Metman, L., Bakay, R. & Corcos, D. [2004]. Effects of deep brain stimulation and medication on bradykinesia and muscle activation in Parkinson's disease, *Brain* 127(3): 491–504.

[52] Vaillancourt, D., Prodoehl, J., Sturman, M., Bakay, R., Metman, L. & Corcos, D. [2006]. Effects of deep brain stimulation and medication on strength, bradykinesia, and electromyographic patterns of the ankle joint in Parkinson's disease, *Mov. Disord.* 21(1): 50–58.

[53] Webber, C. & Zbilut, J. [1994]. Dynamical assessment of physiological systems and states using recurrence plot strategies, *J. Appl. Physiol.* 76(2): 965–973.

[54] Welch, P. [1967]. The used of FFT for estimation of power spectra:a method based on time averaging over short modified periodograms, *IEEE Trans. Audio Electroacoust.* 15: 70–73.

[55] Xia, R. & Rymer, W. [2004]. The role of shortening reaction in mediating rigidity in Parkinson's disease, *Exp. Brain Res.* 156(4): 524–528.

Chapter 7

Distinction of Abnormality of Surgical Operation on the Basis of Surface EMG Signals

Chiharu Ishii

Additional information is available at the end of the chapter

1. Introduction

Recently, minimally invasive surgery such as endoscopic surgery is taking the place of laparotomy. In the field of minimally invasive surgery, a typical commercial surgical robot, such as the da Vinci system produced by Intuitive Surgical Inc., is currently in clinical use. In the robot supported surgery, master-slave system is employed. In such master-slave systems, usually motions of the master device are detected by sensors, and the slave device is controlled to follow the behavior of the master device based on the measured information by those sensors. Therefore, even the mistaken operation will be reflected.

To perform a robotic surgery, a surgeon must have considerable skill. Operation by an unskilled surgeon may result in serious malpractice. Therefore, development of a system which urges an appropriate operation to the unskilled surgeon is in demand. As described in (Tanoue et al., 2007), for training of the robotic surgery, training box or simulator has been generally used.

Recently, in order to help surgeon's dexterity, force feedback to a surgeon through the master device of a surgical robot has been studied in (Ishii et al., 2011). In order to perform safe surgery, (Ikuta et al., 2007) proposed safe operation strategies, called "Safety operation space" and "Variable compliance system" for the surgical robot. The former can prevent collision between the forceps and organs. The latter can reduce the collision force between the forceps and organs.

In addition, training systems to practice operation of surgical robot through simulation using virtual reality environment (e.g. Tokuda et al., 2009), and navigation systems which guide a surgical instrument to the targeted location during the robotic surgery (e.g. Krupa et al., 2003), have been studied.

To the best of our knowledge, however, a system that recognizes and points out any singularity in a surgical operation because of the inexpertness of an unskilled surgeon has not been established yet.

In this study, to detect any singularity in a surgical operation, surface electromyography (SEMG) is employed. Our final goal is to develop such a system that recognizes and points out any singularity in a surgical operation because of the inexpertness of the unskilled surgeon on the basis of operator's SEMG signals during the operation of the surgical robot.

To this end, a novel method for automatic identification of a surgical operation and on-line distinction of any singularity of the identified surgical operation on the basis of the SEMG measurements of an operator and movement of the forceps, is proposed.

Use of the SEMG has attracted an attention of researchers as a method of interaction between human and machines. The amplitude property of waveform and the power spectrum based on frequency analysis are typical information which can be extracted from the SEMG signal.

In (Harada et al., 2010), to control a thumb and index finger of a myoelectric prosthetic hand independently, identification of four finger motions was executed using neural networks on the basis of the SEMG measurements.

In such SEMG based interaction systems, hand gestures are identified by measuring the activities of the musculature system using the SEMG sensors. It is well known that by measuring SEMG signals, not only hand gestures but also distinction between skilled person and unskilled person, and fatigue of the muscle can be recognized (e.g. Sadoyama et al., 1981, and Kizuka et al., 2006).

In (Chen et al., 2007), recognition of 25 kinds of hand gestures consisting of various motions of wrist and fingers, was performed using only two electrodes, and the high recognition rate was successfully obtained. On the other hand, (Nakaya et al., 2010) proposed a hand gesture identification method and a distinction method of any singularity in the identified hand gesture on the basis of the SEMG measurements.

(Kita et al., 2010) proposed a self-organizing approach with level of proficiency to perform stable classification of operation. (Tada et al., 2006) proposed a distinction method of unusual manipulation of a driver when driving an automobile, using the degree of deviation on the basis of the acceleration measurements.

On the other hand, as for the surgical operation, (Hayama et al., 2009) proposed an automatic classification method of four basic surgical operations using a sensing forceps made of a forceps and strain gauges. (Kumagai et al., 2008, and Yamashita, 2009) reported that in surgical operations, a difference arises between skilled surgeon and unskilled surgeon in the following points; the magnitude and direction of the handling force of the object, the manner of having surgical instrument, and surgeon's posture. (Rosen et al., 2006) proposed an evaluation method for the state transition of the forceps operation in cholecystectomy based on comparison of skilled operator and unskilled operator.

In this chapter, a novel method for automatic identification of a surgical operation and on-line distinction of the singularity of the identified surgical operation is proposed. Suturing is divided into six operations. The features of the operation are extracted from the measurements of the movement of the forceps, and then, on the basis of the threshold criteria for the six operations, a surgical operation is identified as one of the six operations.

Next, the features of any singularity of operation are extracted from operator's surface electromyogram signals, and the identified surgical operation is classified as either normal or singular using a self-organizing map: SOM (Kohonen, 2000).

Using the built laparoscopic-surgery simulation box with two forceps, the identification of each surgical operation and the distinction of the singularity of the identified surgical operation were carried out for a specific surgical operation, namely, insertion of a needle during suturing. Each surgical operation in suturing could be identified with more than 80% accuracy, and the singularity of the surgical operation of insertion could be distinguished with approximately 80% accuracy on an average. The experimental results showed the effectiveness of the proposed method.

2. Experimental system

2.1. Simulation box

Laparoscopic-surgery simulation box is shown in Fig.1. Inside of the mannequin, a rubber sheet of 1mm thickness is installed. The image of inside of the simulation box taken by the digital video camera is projected on a central monitor. An operator performs surgical operation using the two forceps, a needle driver (right hand side) and assistant forceps (left hand side) inserted into inside of a mannequin through the trocar, by looking at the monitor. The distance between the two forceps was determined based on the spatial relationship called "triangle formation" recommended in (Hashizume et al., 2005).

In this study, an operator simulates the suturing performed in a laparoscopic surgery using the simulation box.

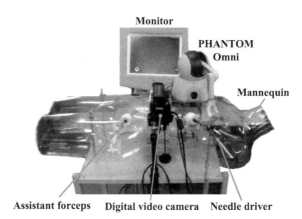

Figure 1. Simulation box

As shown in Fig.2, the movement of the needle driver is measured by the haptics device PHANTOM Omni and attached four strain gauges.

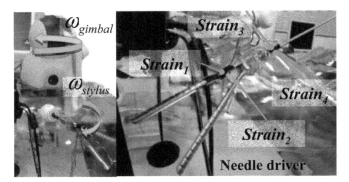

Figure 2. Sensor allocation for needle driver

2.2. Measurement of surface electromyography

The SEMG signals are measured by three electrodes stuck on the forearm of the operator as shown in Fig.3. The electrode 1 was stuck on the musculus flexor carpi radialis, the electrode 2 was stuck on the musculus extensor carpi ulnaris, the electrode 3 was stuck on the musculus extensor carpi radialis longus, and the earth electrode was stuck on the wrist.

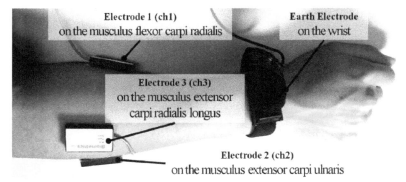

Figure 3. Allocation of surface electrode

3. Distinction of singularity of surgical operation

In this study, suturing is chosen as the objective surgical operation for automatic identification, and especially "insertion of a needle" in suturing is selected as the objective surgical operation for distinction of singularity. The flow for distinction of the singularity of the surgical operation "insertion of a needle" is explained as follows.

3.1. Features of the operation

From measurements of the SEMG signals by three electrodes, the amount of distortion by four strain gauges, and the angular velocity of gimbal and stylus by haptic device, the features are defined as follows.

For identifying the surgical operation, the features of the operation are extracted from the measurements of the movement of the needle driver. Define the features as follows.

$$St_{ch} = \frac{1}{N} \sum_{n=1}^{N} strain_{ch(n)} \tag{1}$$

$$\Omega_{gimbal} = \frac{1}{N} \sum_{n=1}^{N} \omega_{gimbal(n)} \tag{2}$$

$$\Omega_{stylus} = \frac{1}{N} \sum_{n=1}^{N} \omega_{stylusl(n)} \tag{3}$$

where $strain_{ch(n)}$ (ch=1,2...4) is measured value from each strain gauge, $\omega_{gimbal(n)}$ and $\omega_{stylus(n)}$ are measured angular velocity from the haptic device, and n represents the number of the sampled signals.

The features of any singularity of operation are extracted from operator's SEMG signals. The SEMG signals are measured by sampling frequency Fs=2 kHz, and Fast Fourier Transform (FFT) is performed to each SEMG signal for every N=512 sampled data, which is equivalent to perform FFT every 0.256 seconds.

After filtering the SEMG signals by the fourth order Butterworth type band pass filter with 10 Hz to 1 kHz range, the full wave rectification is carried out. In addition, for normalization, the measured SEMG signal of each electrode is divided by the maximum value of the pre-measured SEMG for each operation. Define the features as follows.

Average absolute value: In order to perform pattern recognition, average absolute value of each electrode is often used, which is given as follows.

$$MAV_{ch} = \frac{1}{N} \sum_{n=1}^{N} \left| EMG_{ch(n)} \right| \tag{4}$$

where $EMG_{ch(n)}$ (ch=1,2,3) is SEMG signal of each electrode, and n represents the number of the sampled signals.

Center-of-gravity: In the case where the singular operation is performed, it is expected that change of the waveform can be observed in the SEMG signal. Therefore, as a value representing change of the waveform of the SEMG signal, the value of center-of-gravity is employed, which is defined as follows.

$$cog_{ch} = \sum_{n=1}^{N}\left(n{\cdot}\left|EMG_{ch(n)}\right|\right)\Big/\sum_{n=1}^{N}\left|EMG_{ch(n)}\right| \tag{5}$$

Spectrum ratio: Also, in the case where the singular operation is performed, it is expected that change of distribution of the power spectrum can be observed in the SEMG signal. Therefore, ratio of distribution of the power spectrum of the SEMG signal is also employed.

It is well known that the SEMG signal is distributed in the frequency band between 5 Hz to 500 Hz. Therefore, to see the ratio of the spectrum, frequency band is divided into 5 to 250 Hz and 250 to 500 Hz. Thus, the value of spectrum ratio is defined as follows.

$$Fr_{ch} = Fh_{ch}\big/Fl_{ch} \tag{6}$$

where

$$\begin{cases} Fl_{ch} = \displaystyle\sum_{kf=2}^{N/8}\left|F_{ch(kf)}\right|^{2} & 5 \sim 250Hz \\[2em] Fh_{ch} = \displaystyle\sum_{kf=N/8+1}^{N/4}\left|F_{ch(kf)}\right|^{2} & 250 \sim 500Hz \end{cases} \tag{7}$$

and $|F_{ch(kf)}|$ is spectrum value in frequency kf obtained by Fast Fourier Transform (FFT).

3.2. Automatic identification of surgical operation

The suturing is divided into six operations as shown in Fig.4.

1. Grasping: the grasping state by closing the gripper of the needle driver.
2. Touch: the state where the needle driver touches the objects.
3. Haulage: the state where the needle driver touches the object with grasping the needle disposable.
4. Insertion: the state where the needle disposable is inserted.
5. Extraction: the state where the needle disposable is extracted.
6. Neutral: the state where nothing is operating.

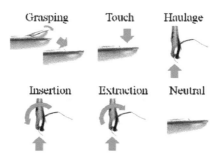

Figure 4. Surgical operations for suturing

In addition, to identify the state of operation of the needle driver using a threshold value, the following new features are defined using the features (1) to (3).

$$V_1 = St_1 \cdot St_2 \tag{8}$$

$$V_2 = \sqrt{St_3^2 + St_4^2} \tag{9}$$

$$V_3 = \Omega_{gimbal} \cdot \Omega_{stylus} \tag{10}$$

For identifying the surgical operation, the following values are defined.

$$T_i = \begin{cases} 1 & V_i > TH_i \\ 0 & else \end{cases}, \quad (i=1,2) \tag{11}$$

$$T_3 = \begin{cases} 1 & (CW) & V_3 > TH_{3H} \\ -1 & (CCW) & V_3 < TH_{3L} \\ 0 & & else \end{cases} \tag{12}$$

where TH_i (i=1,2,3H, 3L) is threshold value for each new feature determined through trial and error. On the basis of the threshold criteria for the six operations, a surgical operation is identified as one of the six operations as shown in Table 1.

Discriminant value /Operation	T₁	T₂	T₃
1.Grasping	1	0	0
2.Touch	0	1	0
3.Haulage	1	1	0
4.Insertion	1	1	1(CW)
5.Extraction	1	1	-1(CCW)
6.Neutral		Else	

Table 1. Logical definition of needle driver operation

3.3. Distinction of singularity of surgical operation

In this study, (a)a normal operation and a (b)singular operation are defined as follows. A normal operation is a surgical operation performed in the expected manner. The singular operation is assumed to be the following surgical operations: (b-1)the surgical operation performed at a posture in which the operator's elbow is raised, denoted as "Posture", (b-2)the surgical operation performed in the state in which the operator is straining, denoted as "Straining", and (b-3)rough surgical operation performed suddenly by the operator, denoted as "Sudden". These are illustrated in Fig.5.

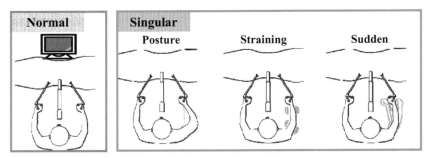

Figure 5. Experimental situations for surgical operation

The surgical operation of (4) insertion of a needle in suturing is classified as either normal or singular by using a self-organizing map: SOM. For classifying the surgical operation, the feature vector which is input to the SOM, is defined as follows using the features (4) to (6).

$$Xs = \left(\frac{MAV_1}{\overline{MAV}}, \frac{MAV_2}{\overline{MAV}}, \frac{MAV_3}{\overline{MAV}}, \frac{cog_2}{cog_1}, \frac{cog_3}{cog_1}, \frac{cog_3}{cog_2}, Fr_1, Fr_2, Fr_3 \right)^T \tag{13}$$

Where $\overline{MAV}$ is an average of MAV_{ch} (ch=1,2,3).

In each state shown in Fig.5, 20 features for normal operation and 60 features for singular operation (20 features for each singular operation) were pre-measured, and total 80 feature vectors defined by (13) are used for batch learning of the SOM. The size of the SOM was determined as hexagon lattice type of 10 x 10.

In addition, k-means method was employed to divide the map into four fields, namely, (a)Normal, (b-1)Posture, (b-2)Straining and (b-3)Sudden.

A feature vector extracted from on-line surgical operation is mapped on the map of the learned SOM, and singular operation is recognized by the distribution on the map. In addition, SOM was built using SOM Toolbox.

4. Experiments and results

The one healthy 20th generation adult man was chosen as an operator, and identification of surgical operation for "suturing" and distinction of the singularity of the identified surgical operation "insertion" were performed.

4.1. Method of experiments

In the experiment, the operator repeatedly performed the suturing process (1) to (6) classified in section 3.2, under the four situations (a)Normal, (b-1)Posture, (b-2)Straining and (b-3)Sudden. The surgical operation "suturing" performed in the experiment is shown in Fig.6. Then, rate of identification of each surgical operation in suturing and rate of distinction of the singularity in the case of (4) insertion were examined.

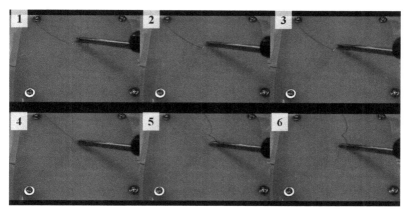

Figure 6. Suturing performed in experiment

4.2. Result for automatic identification

Recognition rate for insertion is shown in Table 2.

A: Actual operation times	19 times
B: Recognition count	21 times
Times which was not counted although operation was performed.	0
Times which was counted although operation was not performed.	2
Difference: |A-B|	2
False recognition rate: |A-B|/A*100	10.5%
Recognition rate	89.5%

Table 2. Recognition rate for insertion operation

Recognition rate for other operations is shown in Table 3.

Operation	A: Actual operation times	B: Recognition count	Recognition rate
1.Grasping	8 times	9 times	87.5%
2.Touch		Non	
3.Haulage	30 times	36 times	80.0%
4.Insertion	19 times	21 times	89.5%
5.Extraction	19 times	22 times	84.2%
6.Neutral	6 times	6 times	100%

Table 3. Recognition rate for automatic identification

The threshold value TH_i (i=1,2,3H, 3L) determined through trial and error is shown in Table 4.

Threshold	Value
TH_1	0.045
TH_2	0.5×10^{-9}
TH_{3H}	0.25
TH_{3L}	0.2

Table 4. Threshold values

As shown in Table 3, each surgical operation could be identified with more than 80% accuracy.

4.3. Result for singularity distinction

In order to classify the singularity of the surgical operation of (4) insertion, a SOM was used. The SOM was constructed by batch learning using the feature vectors of any singularity of operation pre-extracted from SEMG in the case of insertion. Fig.7 shows the constructed SOM and distribution of the mapping of the feature vectors extracted on-line from SEMG for each experimental operation of insertion. The domain of the SOM is roughly divided into two fields, which include the domain for the normal operation denoted as "Normal" and the domain for the singular operation denoted as "Singular." In addition, the domain for the singular operation is divided into three fields, namely, "Posture," "Straining," and "Sudden."

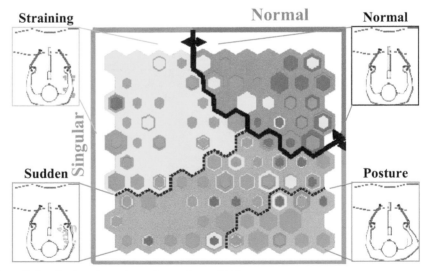

Figure 7. Distribution of experimental operation on SOM

The number of the hexagon counted in each field on the map is shown in Table 5.

	Situation			
	Normal	Posture	Straining	Sudden
Normal field	39	1	14	28
Posture field	2	24	4	7
Straining field	2	20	23	31
Sudden field	8	33	28	23
Total count	51	78	69	89

Table 5. The number of hexagon counted in each field on SOM

Recognition rate for singularity distinction is shown in Table 6.

	Recognition rate[%]	
Normal	76.5	(39/51)
Singular	81.8	(193/236)
Posture	30.8	(24/78)
Straining	33.3	(23/69)
Sudden	25.8	(23/89)

Table 6. Recognition rate for singularity distinction

As shown in Table 5, the normal and the singular operation of insertion could be distinguished with 76.5% and 81.8% accuracy, respectively. However, the accuracy of recognition of the singularity (i.e., "Posture," "Straining," or "Sudden") of the operation is approximately 30%.

As one of the reasons of this low recognition rate in the singularity distinction, the following cause is considered. In the states of "Posture", "Straining" and "Sudden", the singular operation is similar, and the difference does not appear easily in the feature vector.

In order to examine efficiency of each feature, namely average absolute value, center-of-gravity and spectrum ratio, in the feature vector defined by equation (13), singular operation was recognized by SOM using the three-dimensional feature vector which consists of each feature only. Singularity recognition rate for each feature is shown in Table 7.

From Table 7, it turns out that the average absolute value contributes to distinction of normal operation compared with the center-of-gravity and the spectrum ratio, and conversely, the center-of-gravity and the spectrum ratio contribute to the whole singularity distinction compared with the average absolute value.

Based on the above result, to raise the singularity recognition rate in each state (Posture, Straining, and Sudden), singularity distinction was performed repeatedly by combining three kinds of features in the feature vector (Average absolute value, Center-of-gravity, and Spectrum ratio) through trial and error.

As a result, the best singularity recognition rate was obtained for the following six-dimensional feature vector removing the spectrum ratio.

$$Xs = \left(\frac{MAV_1}{MAV}, \frac{MAV_2}{MAV}, \frac{MAV_3}{MAV}, \frac{cog_2}{cog_1}, \frac{cog_3}{cog_1}, \frac{cog_3}{cog_2} \right)^T \qquad (14)$$

Then, two operators were added and the singularity distinction was performed by SOM using the feature vector defined by (14). Recognition rate for singularity distinction using the feature vector given by (14) is shown in Table 8.

	Recognition rate[%]		
	Average absolute value	Center-of-gravity	Spectrum ratio
Normal	76.5	78.4	37.3
Singular	80.9	85.2	84.7
Posture	35.9	24.4	59.0
Straining	42.0	39.1	24.6
Sudden	31.5	30.3	24.7

Table 7. Singularity recognition rate for each feature

	Recognition rate[%]					
	Operator A		Operator B		Operator C	
Normal	76.5	(39/51)	72.0	(36/50)	86.0	(43/50)
Singular	81.4	(192/236)	89.3	(134/150)	72.0	(108/150)
Posture	25.6	(20/78)	74.0	(37/50)	44.0	(22/50)
Straining	31.9	(22/69)	96.0	(48/50)	82.0	(41/50)
Sudden	25.8	(23/89)	56.0	(28/50)	32.0	(16/50)

Table 8. Modified recognition rate for singularity distinction

From Table 8, for the operators B and C, the singularity recognition rate for "Posture" and "Straining" was improved.

5. Conclusion

In this study, a novel method for automatic identification of a surgical operation and on-line distinction of the singularity of the identified surgical operation was proposed. The surgical operation "suturing" was performed using two forceps, namely a needle driver and assistant forceps, in the built simulation box for laparoscopic-surgery. Then, the identification of the surgical operation for "suturing" and the singularity distinction of the identified surgical operation "insertion of a needle" were carried out.

As for the identification of the surgical operation, suturing was divided into six operations. The features of the operation are extracted from the measurements of the movement of the forceps, namely the amount of distortion measured by four strain gauges and the angular velocity of gimbal and stylus measured by haptic device PHANTOM Omni. Then, on the basis of the threshold criteria for the six operations, the surgical operation was identified as one of the six operations. Each surgical operation in suturing could be identified with more than 80% accuracy.

As for the singularity distinction of the identified surgical operation, when the surgical operation was identified as "insertion of a needle", general distinction of normal operation or singular operation and distinction of three kinds of the states, namely "Posture", "Straining" or "Sudden" in the singular operation, were performed by the SOM using the 6-dimensional feature vector which extracted the features from SEMG. Then, the singularity of the surgical operation of insertion could be distinguished with approximately 80% accuracy on an average.

On the other hand, recognition rate of each state in the singular operation was approximately 30% to 90% accuracy depending on the individual difference. Therefore, it is difficult to distinguish three kinds of the states in the singular operation with sufficient accuracy.

However, in a complicated surgical operation such as insertion of a needle, it can be said that general distinction of normal operation or singular operation was able to be recognized with high accuracy.

6. Future directions

In this study, operator for the experiments was only three persons. In order to demonstrate the reliability of the proposed automatic identification and singularity distinction method, it is necessary to perform verification of the proposed method by many operators. However, since SEMG depends on the individuals, it is considered that learning of the SOM for singularity distinction for every operator is required.

In addition, it is also necessary to extend the proposed identification and singularity distinction method for a surgical operation performed with not only a right hand but also both hands. As for this point, we are now applying the proposed identification method to a surgical operation of ligation performed with both hands, and the singularity distinction method to a thread knotting also performed with both hands.

Furthermore, construction of the system to avoid malpractice by presenting recognition of the singular operation to the operator and to provide safe endoscopic-surgery is left as future work.

Author details

Chiharu Ishii
Hosei University, Japan

Acknowledgement

The part of this work was supported by Grant-in-Aid for Scientific Research (23650100). The author thanks Y. Nakaya for his assistance in experimental works.

7. References

Chen, X.; Zhang, X.; Zhao, Z.Y. & Yang, J.H. (2007). Multiple Hand Gesture Recognition based on Surface EMG Signal, *Proceedings of International Conference on Bioinformatics and Biomedical Engineering*, pp. 506-509

Harada, A.; Ishii, C.; Nakakuki, T. & Hikita, M. (2010). Robot Finger Design for Myoelectric Prosthetic Hand and Recognition of Finger Motions via Surface EMG, *Proceedings of 2010 IEEE International Conference on Automation and Logistics*, pp. 273-278

Hashizume, M.; Konishi, K.; Okazaki, K. & Tanoue, K. (2005). Fundamental Training for safe Endoscopic Surgery, Daidogakkan Press (in Japanese)

Hayama, Y.; Kurita, Y.; Kawahara, T.; Okajima, M. & Ogasawara, T. (2009). Automatic Measurement of Forceps Manipulation Logs for Laparoscopic Surgery, Journal of Japan Society of Computer Aided Surgery, Vol.11, No.3, pp. 328-329 (in Japanese)

Ikuta, K.; Hasegawa, M. & Goto, H. (2007). Total System of Hyper Finger for Remote Minimally Invasive Surgery (The 9th Report) Proposal and Experimental Verification of Safety Operation Strategies, *Proceedings of the 16th Annual Meeting of The Japan Society of Computer Aided Surgery*, pp. 43-44

Ishii, C.; Mikami, H.; Nakakuki, T. & Hashimoto, H. (2011). Bilateral Control for Remote Controlled Robotic Forceps System with Time Varying Delay, *Proceedings of IEEE International Conference on Human System Interaction*, pp. 330-335

Kita, K.; Kato, R. & Yokoi, H. (2010). EMG-to-Motion Classification for Prosthetic Applications ? A Self-Organizing Approach with Level of Proficiency -, Journal of the Robotics Society of Japan, Vol.28, No.7, pp. 783-791 (in Japanese)

Kizuka, T.; Masuda, T.; Kiryu, T & Sadoyama, T. (2006). Biomechanism Library Practical Usage of Surface Electromyogram, Tokyo Denki University Press (in Japanese)

Kohonen, T. (2000). Self-Organizing Maps, *Springer*

Krupa, A.; Gangloff, J.; Doignon, C.; de Mathelin, M. F.; Morel, G.; Leroy, J.; Soler, L. & Marescaux, J. (2003). Autonomous 3-D Positioning of Surgical Instruments in Robotized Laparoscopic Surgery Using Visual Servoing, IEEE Transactions on Robotics and Automation, Vol.19, No.5, pp. 842-853

Kumagai, T.; Yamashita, J.; Morikawa, O.; Yokoyama, K.; Fujimaki, S.; Konishi, T.; Ishimasa, H.; Murata, H. & Tomoda. K. (2008). Distance Education System for Teaching Manual Skills in Endoscopic Paranasal Sinus Surgery Using "HyperMirror" Telecommunication Interface, Proceedings of IEEE Virtual Reality 08, pp. 233-236

Nakaya, Y.; Ishii, C.; Nakakuki, T. & Hikita, M. (2010). A Practical Approach for Recognition of Hand Gesture and Distinction of Its Singularity, *Proceedings of 2010 IEEE International Conference on Automation and Logistics*, pp. 474-479

Rosen, J.; Brown, J. D.; Chang, L.; Sinanan, M. N. & Hannaford, B. (2006). Generalized Approach for Modeling Minimally Invasive Surgery as a Stochastic Process Using a Discrete Markov Model, IEEE Transactions on Biomedical Engineering, Vol.53, No.3, pp. 399-413

Sadoyama, T. & Miyano, H. (1981). Frequency analysis of surface EMG to evaluation of muscle fatigue, European Journal of Applied Physiology and Occupational Physiology, Vol.47, No.3, pp. 239-246

Tada, M.; Omura, R.; Naya, F.; Noma, H.; Toriyama, T. & Kogure, K. (2006). Analysis of Steering Control Behavior Using 3D-Accelerometers, IPSJ SIG Technical Report, SIG-CVIM-93, pp. 233-240 (in Japanese)

Tanoue, K. & Hashizume, M. (2007). Advanced medicine and innovative technology, Fukuoka Acta Medica, Vol.98, No.4, pp. 100-105 (in Japanese)

Tokuda, J.; Fischer, G. S.; Papademetris, X.; Yaniv, Z.; Ibanez, L.; Cheng, P.; Liu, H.; Blevins, J.; Arata, J.; Golby, A. J.; Kapur, T.; Pieper, S.; Burdette, E. C.; Fichtinger, G.; Tempany, C. M. & Hata, N. (2009). OpenIGTLink: an open network protocol for image-guided therapy environment, The International Journal of Medical Robotics and Computer Assisted Surgery, Vol.5, No.4, pp. 423-434

Yamashita, J. (2009). A distance- and Self-Education System to Learn Experts' Postures for Technical Skills Training in Endoscopic Sinus Surgery, Journal of Japan Society of Computer Aided Surgery, Vol.11, No.3, pp. 170-171 (in Japanese)

Permissions

The contributors of this book come from diverse backgrounds, making this book a truly international effort. This book will bring forth new frontiers with its revolutionizing research information and detailed analysis of the nascent developments around the world.

We would like to thank Dr. Ganesh R. Naik, for lending his expertise to make the book truly unique. He has played a crucial role in the development of this book. Without his invaluable contribution this book wouldn't have been possible. He has made vital efforts to compile up to date information on the varied aspects of this subject to make this book a valuable addition to the collection of many professionals and students.

This book was conceptualized with the vision of imparting up-to-date information and advanced data in this field. To ensure the same, a matchless editorial board was set up. Every individual on the board went through rigorous rounds of assessment to prove their worth. After which they invested a large part of their time researching and compiling the most relevant data for our readers. Conferences and sessions were held from time to time between the editorial board and the contributing authors to present the data in the most comprehensible form. The editorial team has worked tirelessly to provide valuable and valid information to help people across the globe.

Every chapter published in this book has been scrutinized by our experts. Their significance has been extensively debated. The topics covered herein carry significant findings which will fuel the growth of the discipline. They may even be implemented as practical applications or may be referred to as a beginning point for another development. Chapters in this book were first published by InTech; hereby published with permission under the Creative Commons Attribution License or equivalent.

The editorial board has been involved in producing this book since its inception. They have spent rigorous hours researching and exploring the diverse topics which have resulted in the successful publishing of this book. They have passed on their knowledge of decades through this book. To expedite this challenging task, the publisher supported the team at every step. A small team of assistant editors was also appointed to further simplify the editing procedure and attain best results for the readers.

Our editorial team has been hand-picked from every corner of the world. Their multi-ethnicity adds dynamic inputs to the discussions which result in innovative outcomes. These outcomes are then further discussed with the researchers and contributors who give their valuable feedback and opinion regarding the same. The feedback is then collaborated with the researches and they are edited in a comprehensive manner to aid the understanding of the subject.

Apart from the editorial board, the designing team has also invested a significant amount of their time in understanding the subject and creating the most relevant covers. They scrutinized every image to scout for the most suitable representation of the subject and create an appropriate cover for the book.

The publishing team has been involved in this book since its early stages. They were actively engaged in every process, be it collecting the data, connecting with the contributors or procuring relevant information. The team has been an ardent support to the editorial, designing and production team. Their endless efforts to recruit the best for this project, has resulted in the accomplishment of this book. They are a veteran in the field of academics and their pool of knowledge is as vast as their experience in printing. Their expertise and guidance has proved useful at every step. Their uncompromising quality standards have made this book an exceptional effort. Their encouragement from time to time has been an inspiration for everyone.

The publisher and the editorial board hope that this book will prove to be a valuable piece of knowledge for researchers, students, practitioners and scholars across the globe.

List of Contributors

Mark Halaki
Discipline of Exercise and Sport Science, Faculty of Health Science, The University of Sydney, Sydney, Australia

Karen Ginn
Discipline of Biomedical Sciences, Sydney Medical School, The University of Sydney, Sydney, Australia

Min Lei and Guang Meng
Institute of Vibration, Shock and Noise, State Key Laboratory of Mechanical System and Vibration, Shanghai Jiao Tong University, Shanghai, P R China

Adriano O. Andrade and Alcimar B. Soares
Faculty of Electrical Engineering, Laboratory of Biomedical Engineering, Federal University of Uberlândia, Uberlândia, Brazil

Slawomir J. Nasuto
School of Systems Engineering, University of Reading, Reading, United Kingdom

Peter J. Kyberd
Institute of Biomedical Engineering, University of New Brunswick, Fredericton, Canada

Ryuji Sakakibara, Fuyuki Tateno, Masahiko Kishi and Yohei Tsuyusaki
Neurology, Internal Medicine, Sakura Medical Center, Toho University, Sakura, Japan

Tomoyuki Uchiyama and Tatsuya Yamamoto
Neurology, Chiba University, Chiba, Japan

Tomonori Yamanishi
Urology, Dokkyo Medical College, Tochigi, Japan

Angkoon Phinyomark, Sirinee Thongpanja, Pornchai Phukpattaranont and Chusak Limsakul
Department of Electrical Engineering, Prince of Songkla University, Songkhla, Thailand

Huosheng Hu
School of Computer Science & Electronic Engineering, University of Essex, Colchester, United Kingdom

Rissanen Saara M., Tarvainen Mika P. and Karjalainen Pasi A.
Department of Applied Physics, University of Eastern Finland, Kuopio, Finland

Kankaanpää Markku
Department of Physical and Rehabilitation Medicine, Tampere University Hospital, Tampere, Finland

Chiharu Ishii
Hosei University, Japan

Printed in the USA
CPSIA information can be obtained
at www.ICGtesting.com
JSHW011811301024
72690JS00002B/37